D0457231

THE
Women'sHealth
BDY
CLOCK
DIET

The 6-Week Plan to Reboot Your Metabolism and Lose Weight Naturally

LAURA CIPULLO, RD

RODALE.

RODALE *wellness*

Live happy. Be healthy. Get inspired.

Sign up today to get exclusive access to our authors, exclusive bonuses, and the most authoritative, useful, and cutting-edge information on health, wellness, fitness, and living your life to the fullest.

Visit us online at RodaleWellness.com
Join us at RodaleWellness.com/Join

Rodale books may be purchased for business or promotional use or for special sales. For information, please write to:

Special Markets Department, Rodale Inc., 733 Third Avenue, New York, NY 10017

Women's Health is a registered trademark of Rodale Inc.

Printed in the United States of America

Rodale Inc. makes every effort to use acid-free ♾, recycled paper ♻.

Photographs by Beth Bischoff

Illustration, p. 20, © iStock

Book design by Christina Gaugler

Library of Congress Cataloging-in-Publication Data is on file with the publisher.

ISBN 978–1–62336–658–2 trade hardcover

Distributed to the trade by Macmillan

2 4 6 8 10 9 7 5 3 1 hardcover

We inspire and enable people to improve their lives and the world around them.
rodalebooks.com

To my balance buddies and partners in the kitchen:
my husband, Robert; my sons, Robert and William;
and, of course, all my amazing clients.
You all remind me that personal relationships
are synergistic just like foods in our bodies.

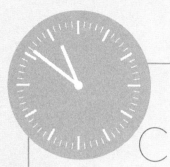

CONTENTS

PART III: BODY CLOCK REPAIR and MAINTENANCE

INTRODUCTION

Timing Is Everything

Reboot your circadian rhythm
for natural weight loss and better health

Imagine feeling calm, wonderful, and happy. Your body is lean, strong, and nimble. It moves with power and grace. You have the energy to accomplish all the tasks of your day, stress-free, with energy to spare. You work hard and play hard, and at the end of the day you fall into bed tired. Not exhausted, but "good tired." You've known that feeling: It's the kind of feel-good exhaustion that welcomes sleep as you drift off to restful slumber for the night.

This is not science fiction. This can actually be your life. In fact, it should be! This is how our bodies were designed to perform, aligned with a natural rhythm governed mostly by the rising and setting sun. This rhythmic ebb and flow of waking and sleeping is an organic cycle that promotes optimal health; it only *seems* like fantasy because this kind of perfection is so terribly far from the life most of us experience. The *Women's Health* Body Clock Diet is designed to reset your body's internal timers to transport you back into a healthier rhythm. It's going to feel great! And you're going to feel good about yourself 24/7 when you've completed this program.

I am so happy you joined the editors at *Women's Health* and me on this journey! You will finally find clarity and enlightenment about what it takes to lose weight naturally, without struggle, and keep it off. Let's face reality: With a plethora of nutrition information from the media to supposed weight-loss gurus to the pages of research, we are dazed and confused by the contradictory claims. How do we know what works for you, me, and even our children? Well, with almost 20 years of clinical nutrition experience as a registered dietitian, I believe I have the answers and the evidence to help you free yourself from the dieting mentality and be truly healthy.

YOUR INTERNAL CLOCK

The goal of this book is to reset your circadian rhythm, the body's 24-hour master clock, and other internal clocks—a harmony of biological rhythms that control sleeping and waking, hunger and fullness hormones, body temperature, blood pressure, digestion, and energy, all of which affect your body composition.

When your body clock is ticking optimally, weight loss and weight maintenance come much more easily because you can allow your natural hunger patterns to guide your food choices and amounts. You don't fall prey to terrible cravings. You don't have to count calories and can adopt my philosophy that "all foods fit" into healthy nutrition. Yes, that means you can literally have your cake and eat it too. Cake! That may sound crazy coming from a certified diabetes educator, but consider this: I am also a certified eating disorders specialist and registered dietitian. I've successfully treated women with extreme binge-eating problems and the "all foods fit" idea works for them, too. So trust me when I say that you don't have to count calories anymore! In fact, counting calories can actually work against you, as I'll demonstrate.

You see, good nutrition is not *just* a numbers game. It's about nurturing your mind, body, and spirit to realign with your natural biorhythms.

NATURE VERSUS NANOTECHNOLOGY

We have a significant challenge with obesity in the country, and in the majority of cases, it's caused by lifestyle hiccups that shift our bodies out of their natural rhythms of waking, eating, being active, and sleeping. The human body has not caught up with the progression of industrialization, technology, and urban life. We're still the same beings that, in the days before iPhones or even windup alarm clocks, woke up with the sun. We weren't built with battery packs to run day and night like robots. Only the Energizer Bunny can keep going and going.

People want to get back to a lifestyle driven by nature versus nanotechnology. However, the answer is not just to turn off your wrist phone and computer. The solution is to reset your master body clock to flow with the rhythm of the 24-hour cycle of light and dark. You know as well as I do that this modern world is not about going with the flow. It's like a race to be the best in which the course isn't linear with a start and finish; instead it can feel more like the exercise wheel in a gerbil's cage, constantly spinning but going nowhere. It's time to get off that crazy wheel.

I COME FROM A BIG ITALIAN FAMILY

My name is Cipullo, which is a derivative of *onion* in Italian. Like an onion, I have a lot of layers you can't see. You do too; we're all complex beings with many layers. Looking at me, the nutritionist, you might be surprised to learn that I used to have an unhealthy relationship with food and that almost everyone in my family is obese. My family members have struggled with their weight—and their health—for many years. My two wonderful uncles, Dennis and Gene, passed away from complications of poor self-care, including the serious medical problems associated with diabetes. I grew up in a home that looked like the one in *The Sopranos,* minus the Mafia. The men in my family were 300 pounds plus, a diabetes diagnosis was the norm, and large portions of food were always within a fork's reach. Here's a telling picture: At holidays, my mom would make 30 pounds of potatoes for 15 people!

I learned about registered dietitians and their work through my uncles' health struggles. Uncle Gene allowed me to join his nutrition session with his dietitian when I was just a sophomore in high school. That experience convinced me to pursue human nutrition and dietetics. After earning my RD, my uncle Dennis was diagnosed with diabetes and related medical complications. His doctor knew I was a registered dietitian and asked me to write a medical nutrition plan for Uncle Dennis as a test. If I got it right, Dr. Pattner promised to refer clients to me. Well, he liked my plan and started referring clients. I felt great satisfaction trying to help my uncle and others to eat healthier. I know that successful weight loss can happen through lifestyle changes, but I'm also realistic about how hard it can be to change lifelong habits.

The women in my family are mostly apple shaped. When I was growing up, my mom had a magnet on our refrigerator that read "Joan, don't break your diet." I found that quite ironic. Weight management was always top of mind among the Cipullos, yet the adults were all overweight and in poor health. I grew up hearing the greeting "Hi, you look like you lost weight" or "Happy Thanksgiving, you gained weight." Um, WTF?

Through my family, I learned firsthand what didn't work. While I was never "heavy," I did struggle through high school and college to find a healthy relationship with food and body image. I got caught up in the throes of weighing myself daily, trying to control the number on the scale, and running miles and miles to compensate for what I ate. Food and my body ruled my thoughts for a long time.

I was determined to be healthy, and by that I mean balanced. I set out on a mission to learn how to eat for weight loss and maintenance and then to share the message. I learned that delicious food, including steak and Uncle Dennis's Italian pastries, can be part of a healthy lifestyle with a fit body when eaten in moderation to satisfy true physical hunger. But I also learned how impossibly hard it is to change the habits of someone who doesn't want to change. Dietitians and books like this one are only worthy of your time if you're willing to implement their advice. You can do this, I know you can, but you must want to in your heart of hearts.

YOUR TOTAL BODY CLOCK TRANSFORMATION

My cousin Andrea always jokes that I should put a picture of our family on my office door to let clients know that I come from a tribe of meat and pasta eaters, not skinny vegetarians, and that I understand firsthand the health implications of an excessive diet and sedentary lifestyle. It would also illustrate the fact that your genetics and the environment in which you were raised do not condemn you to a life of poor health. I grew up in a family of unhealthy eaters, and yet I was able to change my lifestyle to become a fit foodie. And you will, too. Good health is possible for anyone.

Note that I'm focusing on the word *health* and not *weight*. One of the most important lessons you will learn in this book is to forget about the number on the scale. We will use the word *weight* for clarity, but I want you to try hard to stop identifying yourself by your pound weight. I'm convinced that the relentless obsession with number of pounds actually prevents weight loss. What's the first thing that happens when you visit your doctor after handing in your insurance card? The nurse weighs you. Most doctors take that scale number and plug it into a height-weight chart that shows your body mass index (BMI). BMI, based on your height and weight, is an inaccurate measure of body fat and overall health because it doesn't take into account bone density, muscle mass, and racial and sex differences. Frankly, I think BMI is BS. It's a useless tool for gauging one's health, and it's often misleading. For example, in a new study, researchers from Oxford Brookes University in the United Kingdom found that more than a third of 3,000 people who were classified as having a normal, healthy BMI were actually at risk for obesity-related problems like cardiovascular disease. BMI may have given them a false sense of security when it should have made them aware of potential health risks.

In my private practice, the scale remains hidden. I want my clients to ignore the number of pounds or the BMI and use how they feel as a gauge of mind, body, and health. Want a more accurate tool than your bathroom scale? Try the 10-second string test on page 13.

My friend, you are not alone in your quest for balance, weight loss, and health. We've all been there. In this book you will hear stories from my clients about how they choose to eat all foods, accept their bodies as they are, and even lose weight. I hope they will inspire you to adopt a neutral food and body language focusing on the positives.

This book is about working synergistically with your body clock to lose weight naturally. You'll learn that you absolutely must eat enough food to prevent a decrease in your metabolism. Restrictive diets (also called starvation diets) can slow your metabolism by as much as 30 percent, disrupting your body clock and sabotaging your weight-loss hopes. The *Women's Health* Body Clock Diet meal structures will help you to actually boost your metabolism, not stifle it. You will learn that stress hormones trigger the storage of fat in your cells, and you'll find out how mindfulness and self-compassion are the keys to resetting your body clock into a natural rhythm that promotes a healthy weight.

BENEFITS OF A CLOCK THAT KEEPS TIME

If you truly desire a fresh start with food, mood, and body, let's get started. Over the course of 6 weeks, the Body Clock Diet program will help you to . . .

REVERSE unhealthy habits.

OVERCOME stress.

INCREASE your metabolism to help you burn more calories.

REDUCE your waist circumference (and pass the string test!).

EAT ANYTHING you desire, mindfully.

NEVER COUNT calories again.

HONOR your body and mind.

LOSE weight and feel great.

BE HAPPY with the person you are now!

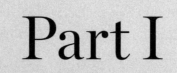

Part I

HOW
YOU
TICK

CHAPTER 1

The Dirty Secret about Diets

THEY DON'T WORK. SO LET'S TRY HABITUAL NOURISHMENT INSTEAD. IT'S DELICIOUS AND FUN!

For years dietitians and doctors could not explain why some clients easily lose weight, while others are only able to stop weight gain—and they struggle to do even that! In my world, I always knew fad diets didn't work, but what does work?

Through years of improving clients' eating habits and their health, I have observed that those who don't get hung up on tracking the numbers on the bathroom scale are able to lose weight more easily and keep it off as compared to people who obsess over the fluctuations of a pound gained here, a pound lost there. Research is finally available to support what I've always thought: Strict dieting usually yields the opposite of the desired effect.

Research shows that any restrictive diet can deliver success—for a time. High-carb, low-fat diets prove just as successful as the low-carb, high-protein diets that are currently in vogue. In the end, people lose weight from any diet that reduces calories consumed, but the tendency is to go off the diet because it proves too difficult to sustain and actually gain more weight than before. You've witnessed this if you keep up with celebrity news. Consider Kirstie Alley, who regained the more than 70 pounds she lost on Jenny Craig. How many other roller-coaster-diet celebs can you recall? Janet Jackson, Kelly Clarkson, Maureen "Marcia Brady" McCormick . . . This is yo-yo dieting; it's not only frustrating and ineffective, it can be dangerous.

You've heard this statistic before? Eighty percent of people who have lost weight on a diet regain it within 2 years. Well, it turns out that the news is even worse than that. A study reported in the journal *Obesity* found that people who followed a very low-calorie diet not only regained their weight but also put on significantly *more* weight than those dieters who followed a less-restrictive plan. And the proof doesn't come from just one source. Researchers at the University of California at Los Angeles analyzed 31 long-term diet studies and found that about two-thirds of dieters regained more weight within 4 or 5 years than they initially lost.

But this news shouldn't bum you out. On the contrary, it points to something very positive: Eat! Our culture of instant gratification, i.e., quick weight loss, says starve your body to lose weight fast, but the science shows that doesn't work! And there is a better way.

BECCA DID IT, AND SO CAN YOU

I live and breathe everything I teach in my practice, but sometimes clients just don't have faith that my positive approach to nutrition will result in weight loss. I understand their doubt; they've been programmed to think diet, diet, diet. Here's an example.

Not long ago a young woman named Heather came into the office obviously frustrated. She said she had not seen any significant changes in her body, and she wanted to quit my program. At our first appointment together, Heather warned me that she wanted to see physical results. "I want to change my relationship with food, but I really want to be thin again," she said. "I tend to stop something within a week if I don't see results." I encouraged her to give it time, because lasting change does not come overnight.

Heather hated her body. She would not date or even go to dinner with friends because her shape embarrassed her. "I'm giving up," she told me. "In the past few weeks I've started to go back to my old habits. I'm making the choice to eat for emotional reasons. I know this doesn't help, but I'm helpless." By the way, Heather is by no means helpless, and she's not lazy. She loves to exercise: She does spinning twice a week and both yoga and kickboxing once weekly. And she felt even more frustrated because she believed her exercise hadn't made a dent in her weight.

I sympathized with Heather and validated her feelings. Then I told her the story of Becca, a client I had seen earlier in the week. Several years ago, Becca came to my New Jersey office while she was home from college on summer break. She had gained about 30 pounds at school and was trying to lose this weight on her own, but nothing worked. She asked me to put her on a very low-calorie diet. I explained that I didn't recommend low-calorie diets because calorie restriction often leads to bingeing. I showed her research that suggests that women who restrict calories during the day typically end up bingeing at night on even more calories than they would have consumed in an entire day if they had simply eaten normally throughout the day.

Becca, like so many dieters, kept calories to a minimum during the day in an effort to "be good." By the time night fell, she became ravenous and fatigued. She felt out of control upon taking her first bite of food and literally couldn't stop eating because her body was truly hungry, maybe even starving. Her body, like everyone's, is biologically set up for survival. When it thinks it's starving, it craves calories and hoards them as fat out of sheer will to survive.

After the high-calorie binge, the guilt came tumbling down. Becca labeled herself as "bad" because she ate more than she planned and felt undisciplined and weak; she vowed that this would be the last night she let food control her. Tomorrow she would be strong. Every cell in Becca's body was dialed into deprivation mode; her body felt it must hoard as many calories as possible now to survive, for tomorrow there might be no food. Not only is this an awful way to go through life, but this binge/restrict cycle also typically results in a 30 percent decrease in resting metabolism, causing the body to function at only 70 percent capacity and thus burn fewer calories.

I explained to Heather that Becca's obsession with the scale and monitoring every morsel of food was sabotaging her goals. It was screwing up her body clock, big-time.

A WEIGHTY SUBJECT: CHRONOBIOLOGY

You can't see them, but deep within every cell of your body are tiny time-pieces that drive many of your critical biological functions like body temperature, heart rate, blood pressure, hormones, hunger, digestion, fatigue, and alertness.

When we talk about *body clock*, we really mean circadian rhythm, those physical, mental, and behavioral patterns that occur in our bodies during a daily 24-hour cycle of light and dark. The study of these circadian rhythms is called chronobiology, and it's a booming field as new research continues to show how great an influence your body clock exerts on your health and even your waist. It's even more important to your body weight than your metabolism or the amount of calories and dietary fat you consume. You'll read more about how this works in Chapter 3.

There are many tiny peripheral clocks all over your body, and they're all governed by a master body clock, which is called the suprachiasmatic nucleus and is located in your brain's hypothalamus. That's a mouthful, I know, so let's call it the SCN spot. This powerful bit of tissue is made up of about 20,000 nerve cells. The SCN sets a 24-hour timing system that helps your body to anticipate changes such as when you are going to sleep, wake, eat, and digest.

One huge role of the SCN, for example, is controlling the production of melatonin, the hormone that makes you sleepy. Located very near the optic nerves that relay intel from the eyes to the brain, the SCN cells are highly influenced by light entering your eyeballs. When the sun sets and there's less light tickling your SCN, more melatonin is produced. But say you stay up late bathed in overhead lighting and the blue light of your computer screen while you surf the web and enjoy a rum and Coke. The light and booze buzz can knock your poor master body clock out of sync. The result: It's sort of like a bad case of jet lag without the benefit of visiting Paris. And weight gain without the pleasure of buttery croissants!

I told Heather that Becca, after another failed diet attempt, finally saw the light. She turned up in my Manhattan office. "You were right," she said. "I'm ready to listen to whatever you tell me to do."

I let Becca's statement sink in with Heather, and then I continued to tell her the rest of Becca's story.

After a hug, Becca and I created a new meal structure to help reset her mind-set and her body clock. I suggested Becca start with three meal options for breakfast, lunch, and dinner, then five snack options that she could choose from twice a day. For her part, Becca agreed to stop weighing herself daily.

Note that I used the word *structure*, not meal *plan*. I prefer the term *structure* because it's a foundation on which to build, not an absolute plan set in stone that you must follow without deviation. I prefer an outline to guide meal decisions instead of a strict menu of eat only this and not that. We want to steer clear of the black-and-white, good-versus-bad attitude of adherence to a strict plan, because it starts to resemble the restrictive diets that destroy natural biorhythms.

Since Heather was fixated on weighing herself, as Becca was, I proceeded to show her how Becca's weight came off slowly and explained how even a year and a half later, she was still losing weight. I wanted to make the point to Heather that lasting weight loss doesn't mean instant weight loss, so she shouldn't expect super-fast results and lose faith. Until her body clock reset into a natural, healthy rhythm, Becca's body would still operate on alert mode, fearful of further restriction and holding on to calories. When her body realized it was no longer going to be restricted, the weight came off much more dramatically and rapidly.

The best part is that Becca could just keep doing what she was doing. There's no diet plan per se to drop from, to "fail." She no longer binges and is no longer controlled by food. She often joins her friends at happy hour and doesn't feel guilty about the indulgence when she gets home. In time, her body will get to its "set weight," that is, her natural, ideal, healthy weight, and Becca will not need to change anything to maintain it. She will have reached that sweet spot of total body clock balance. And it will feel good.

That's the goal for you too!

Heather got the message. I put Becca's chart away and asked Heather to jot down three simple self-care goals she would like to work on before our next session.

Heather wrote:

1. Eat one social meal with friends per day (she had been avoiding doing this due to her embarrassment with her current weight).

2. Practice relaxation breathing techniques before one meal daily.

3. Read a book about reversing diabetes with diet. (Heather brought her blood work in to my office; it revealed she had elevated hemoglobin A1C, a measure of average blood sugar over 3 months. Her numbers showed that she had prediabetes, the precursor to full-blown insulin resistance, or type 2 diabetes. We will learn more about the dangers of high blood sugar later.)

Heather made the shift, and she is currently doing well, resetting her body clock and losing pounds.

Becca did it. I've done it. And you are about to do it. Reset your body clock and let your body work for you. Get started by following these three steps.

RECOMMENDATION 1: Make sure to avoid extreme dieting.

RECOMMENDATION 2: Retrain your brain to understand that diet is defined as habitual nourishment. Yes, that's the way *Webster's Dictionary* defines it. The most important thing you can do for yourself is understand that the *Women's Health* Body Clock Diet is your opportunity to erase years of fad diets and a broken metabolism and get yourself on a schedule of patterned eating where all foods fit. No struggle. No sacrifice. Just a clock that keeps your body in balance naturally.

RECOMMENDATION 3: Just as Heather did, take a few minutes now to write down three self-care goals and how you hope to nurture yourself in the next 6 weeks. Losing 30 pounds is not a goal. That is self-sabotage. Focus on positive change in your mind and body as a goal; for example, "to feel comfortable in my body as I walk down the street" or "to be able to eat cake without feeling guilty." Search your soul and start writing.

1. _____

2. _____

3. _____

Nine Lessons *for* Leaner Living

HELPFUL NOTES TO DECONSTRUCT THE NEGATIVITY AROUND YOUR WEIGHT

Weight gain. Inability to lose pounds. Skinny jeans that must have shrunk, because we just can't squeeze into them any longer! Hey, we've all been down that road, so let's take a detour.

It's not your fault! Remember my clients Becca and Heather? Stop beating yourself up the way they did. Be kind to yourself, because you are your own best friend. Recognize that your weight is not the result of a flaw in your character; it's not caused by something you did wrong. Being wide in the waist and out of shape is a result of something much greater than the piece of peanut butter chocolate cake you ate last night. It's the result of a biological body clock that has not adapted to the excesses of food everywhere, emotional stress, and the mad pace of our modern world. So shed the guilt and gain the knowledge. When you stop blaming yourself, you begin to see that you're worthy of the self-care you need to establish through a new routine.

STOP THE DIETING MENTALITY!

Did you know that Americans spend $60 billion annually on diets, diet foods, and weight-loss remedies? The diet industry is pervasive, and we're all falling prey to it because it's impossible to avoid the constant drumbeat of "you're fat and you need help" messages. We need an obesity epidemic cleanse.

Let's start by deconstructing the negative thoughts surrounding our food and our bodies. Read through the following nine statements. Have you ever spoken these words? Circle each statement below that resonates with you.

1. "I know what to eat, but I just can't do it."

2. "On a good day I eat . . . but on a bad day I eat . . . !"

3. "That skinny bitch . . . I'm so jealous. She can eat whatever she wants, and I just look at food and gain weight."

4. "No matter what I do, the scale never goes down."

5. "I lost 40 pounds on Jenny Craig, but I gained it all back and more."

6. "Tonight is my birthday, and we're going out to eat. I'll start my diet tomorrow."

7. "You look so good; what are you eating?"

8. "My sister got the good genes, and I got the bad genes."

9. "I could look like her, but I don't want to eat bird food."

Familiar words, huh? Most American women have spoken those phrases or at least heard other women say them. Let's dig a little deeper into those nine statements and apply lessons to each that will help you overcome the pervasive negativity surrounding food and weight.

Statement 1
"I know what to eat, but I just can't do it."

Many people tell me they know more about nutrition than I do or they know what to do, but they just don't do it. Well, bah, humbug! Who really knows how to eat, what to eat, and when to eat? Our parents definitely did *not* teach us this one. More than half of them don't have a positive relationship with food. If someone really knew how to eat, what to eat, and when to eat, they would know that eating is more than just fueling your body. It's about enjoyment and fun. It encompasses mind, body, and spirit. Nothing in this world works alone; every little atom affects every other. Remember, we're like onions—we have many layers. And so does our food.

LESSON 1

Our mind, body, and spirit are one. How we feel about our food, as much as the food we eat, affects our "one."

Statement 2
"On a good day I eat good food, such as proteins, fruits, and vegetables, but on a bad day I eat bad food—you know, carbs—bread, pasta, and sweets."

When did food become a value judgment? Why does what we eat determine if we are going to have a good day or bad day? Why does getting on the scale determine a good day with good spirits versus a bad day with mood swings? I'm not sure who came up with this notion, but throw it away. It's useless, and it sabotages all efforts to reset your body clock. When we refer to body clock, please remember: Your body clock is mind, body, and spirit. I'm telling you now: There are no good foods or bad foods. Stop judging them by giving them labels. Just as there are no good kids or bad kids, just kids who behave badly at times, foods should be identified fairly, too. Granted, it's hard to break the labeling mind-set, but you must.

LESSON 2

Stop labeling food with morals and values. Start identifying food by its name. Food is food. An apple is an apple and a cupcake is a cupcake. And a scoop of "death by chocolate" has never murdered anyone, so why call it "bad"?

Statement 3
"That skinny bitch . . . I'm so jealous. She can eat whatever she wants, and I just look at food and gain weight."

Here's a classic! Who hasn't said or heard this before? Finger-pointing, blame, jealousy, competition, and worse, hating yourself for being hungry—all negatives. Isn't that a sad way to go through life? But there's another way, which requires a shift in attitude that can be life changing. Have you heard of the self-care and self-compassion movement? (Read more about it in Chapter 10.) This psychological and behavioral approach is going to be one of the keys to your success.

LESSON 3

Stop stressing and start smiling. Whenever a negative thought enters your mind, find a way to sweep it away by being positive and proactive.

Statement 4
"No matter what I do, the scale never goes down."

How frustrating is this one? How depressing is it to go to your doctor's office, hear your weight, and be told you're obese according to the body mass index (BMI) chart. "I'd like you to start eating healthy and lose at least 50 pounds," your doctor says. "Have a good day. Next!"

Well, that wasn't helpful. You think, *I'm trying, but nothing works. I hate the scale and I hate you, doc.* Let's get one thing straight—health is not weight. They are not synonymous. Weight is just one of many measurements, including lab values such

SLEEP OFF MORE POUNDS

Did you know that more than 50 percent of daily fat loss occurs while you're sleeping? I hope that puts the importance of sleep and maintaining an "on-time" body clock into perspective for keeping a healthy body.

Dozens of recent research studies have shown that high-quality sleep and maintaining a regular sleep routine correlate with lower body fat. One particular trial followed 245 overweight women ages 35 to 55 who were involved in a weight-loss program. The study's researchers reported in a 2012 issue of the journal *Obesity* that getting good-quality slumber and more than 7 hours of sleep per night increased the likelihood of weight-loss success by 33 percent.

Are you ready to start singing lullabies to yourself tonight?

THE STRING TEST
Find Out If Your Waist Is Healthy in Just 10 Seconds

A much better way to get a ballpark evaluation of your weight and health than BMI or even your bathroom scale is the string test. Cut a piece of string to the length of your height, then fold it in half and wrap it around your waist. If the ends overlap, your waist size is less than half your height—the ideal range. Snug string? That could indicate that you're carrying more belly fat than is healthy for your size.

as triglycerides, glucose, and C-reactive protein; behaviors such as exercise and sleep cycles; and more that can help assess one's true health status and risk of cardiovascular disease, diabetes, and even eating disorders.

I don't like weight scales. They don't accurately gauge health or percent of body fat. The specific number on the scale reflects just a moment in time. It's the trend of those numbers and how quickly the numbers fluctuate that may provide insight into your health status. Remember that losing too much weight can be just as unhealthy as gaining too much weight too quickly. For example, I have clients who are considered obese with a BMI over 30 but are much healthier than clients with a BMI under 20. Why? Because it's not just about the number, but what you do to get there. Starving yourself or drinking wine instead of eating meals to get yourself to a low scale number is not healthy. I'd much rather see a client eat a balanced diet, exercise often, and weigh more.

The scale also provides a "score," yet another unfair evaluation of one's worth as a human being if the score isn't trending in the direction one hopes. It can make you feel lazy and unattractive—like a loser. Hopping on the scale can be akin to a daily put-down from a bully. But the bully is you.

LESSON 4

Health and happiness matter more than the number on the scale. Feel confident and celebrate yourself the way you are. Be your own best friend. Forget the scale and focus on eating well, moving often, and being mindful of the many gifts and talents you share with the world, which is your real worth as a human being.

Statement 5
"I lost 40 pounds on Jenny Craig, but I gained it all back and more."

How many diets have you tried? Atkins, Weight Watchers, Nutrisystem, the Cabbage Soup Diet, the Scarsdale Diet, the BluePrint juice cleanse, and now this, the Body Clock Diet. Don't worry. This is not a fad diet. This is the anti-diet. A fad diet has a beginning and an end point. And once you stop your fad diet, you tend to overeat and gain all the weight back plus more. This happens every time you choose a calorie-restrictive diet, so you end up with a higher set weight than if you had never restricted in the first place. This can lead to an unhealthy pattern called yo-yo dieting. (See "How Dieting Puts on the Pounds.") I want you to start thinking about the Body Clock Diet as a natural, habitual pattern of eating at regular intervals that will help to bring your body into healthy harmony.

LESSON 5
Starving yourself ultimately makes you fatter. Stop dieting and establish a lifestyle habit of eating well.

Statement 6
"Tonight is my birthday, and we're going out to eat. I'll start my diet tomorrow."

This classic declaration is a sure way to set yourself up for failure. The idea of starting a diet tomorrow rather than choosing to create change right now is the MO of start/stop fad dieting. Self-care is not a game that begins and ends. Habitual nourishment means establishing a pattern of eating with no right or wrong, winning or losing. Food, exercise, and self-care are choices we make. There is no cheating—only choices with consequences. Take a mindful breath, decide to eat or not to eat, and then move on. The cheating mentality is self-sabotaging. Who are you cheating? Yourself?

LESSON 6
All foods fit, and it's about choosing which foods, how much, and when to eat. This is not a game, so cheating is not in your vocabulary.

HOW DIETING PUTS ON THE POUNDS

Typically, when you go on a restrictive diet, you first lose water weight, especially if it's a very low-carbohydrate diet. You store 4 grams of water for every gram of carbohydrate (stored as glycogen) in your body. When you cut the carbs, you lose the water and become dehydrated (and prone to headaches and constipation). Nice, right?

Next, without adequate glycogen for fuel, a couple of things happen: First, your basal metabolic rate (the number of calories your body burns at rest) decreases by 25 to 30 percent to conserve energy, and your brain starts tapping ketones from protein for power. Second, your body sucks up fatty acids for energy, and if you continue to deprive yourself of carbohydrates, your body will attack your muscles (protein in storage) for fuel. This is muscle wasting. Your body is literally consuming its skeletal muscle to survive. Having less muscle on your frame means your metabolism slows even more. It slips into survival mode, conserving energy to keep you alive. This is helpful during a famine or if you're lost in the wilderness without food for weeks. It's not good when the calorie restriction is self-inflicted.

By the way, while muscle wastes, your number of fat cells doesn't decrease. The cells simply shrink. This is an important fact to keep in mind. Because when the rescue team arrives with rations or you go off your restrictive diet at an all-you-can-eat buffet, the influx of calories causes a rapid increase in fat storage. Your metabolism is still in slo-mo mode and can't metabolize the food you're overeating. As a result, those shriveled fat cells balloon, causing fast weight gain, and your belly becomes bigger than it was before.

But that's not the worst of it. A pattern of this kind of weight cycling and yo-yo dieting can actually be more hazardous to your health than a steady increase in weight over time. Studies involving women have shown that frequent yo-yo dieting places them at greater risk of heart disease and may even damage blood vessels and heart tissue.

Statement 7
"You look so good; what are you eating?"

Why are we always connecting appearance to some diet or eating strategy? Perhaps she looks so good because she's happy or is wearing a new outfit or just read an uplifting text from a good friend. Our culture is obsessed with external judgment, external measurements, and everyone else's business. How about reframing that question to "How are you? You look fabulous!" Or "How are you? You seem so happy!" By thinking about someone's behavior, mood, and wellness, you'll stop engaging in the social stigma around appearance and weight. This will in turn help you to live in an easier, kinder world that is concerned with people on an emotional level, not just a physical level.

LESSON 7

Focus on the wellness of the whole person. Ask "How are you?" rather than "How much weight have you lost or gained?"

Statement 8
"My sister got the good genes, and I got the bad genes."

Genetics are definitely part of the picture that affects our health, our biological disposition, and even our temperament. However, we are now learning that our genes are not set in stone. You can turn certain genes on and off through environmental cues and behaviors. The rhythm of your body clock can influence the expression of your genes.

Three Attitude-Shifting Mantras

Choose your favorite and repeat every hour on the hour until it's not fun anymore or you believe these words with all your heart!

1. The New Perfect Is Being Imperfect.

2. Health Is Happiness.

3. Strong Is the New Skinny.

QUIT THE CLEAN-YOUR-PLATE CLUB

Did your parents guilt you into licking your plate clean because "there are starving children overseas who would love your leftovers"? Rid yourself of the clean-your-plate mentality that many of us grew up with. We live in a society where food is overly plentiful and, if anything, we have to make far too many food decisions every day due to this excess. Know you can eat again and know you can eat cake or pizza for breakfast if that helps you to eat less at dinner or dessert. I swear this helps. Start thinking this way now: Leave something on your plate. Stop eating when you're no longer hungry. *How much food you consume counts far more than what food you consume.* Instead of getting bogged down in an eat this, not that mentality, simply make smaller portions a habit.

LESSON 8

Work with your body to create wellness. Don't play the genes card; it's a cop-out.

Statement 9
"I could look like her, but I don't want to eat bird food."

Fruits, vegetables, granola, nuts, whole grains, wheat germ, and even dark chocolate all used to be considered "bird food" or "diet food." We gave them a label, called them things we should be eating more of, and as a result made these foods seem unappealing. But look at what happens when you adopt the attitude that all foods can fit into a healthy diet. Suddenly all foods become appealing. Nothing is sacrificed, so there's no stress. By being mindful of the nutrients in your meals (protein, fat, and carbohydrates), you can choose foods and portion sizes consistent with your metabolic needs, all the while eating cookies and milk!

LESSON 9

All foods fit. Eat nutrient-dense foods 75 percent of the time and less nutrient-dense foods the other 25 percent of the time.

CHAPTER
3

Girls Got Rhythm

UNDERSTANDING YOUR BODY CLOCK AND THE "ZEITGEBERS" THAT MAKE IT CUCKOO

L ong, long, long before Lennon, Harrison, and McCartney penned the lyrics for "Here Comes the Sun," the human organism was shaped by the day-and-night, light-and-dark cycle created by the daily rotation of the Earth around the sun. This 24-hour, 360-degree spin influences biological timers deep in the core of our bodies—what we refer to as our body clocks. Our body clocks respond to shifts in our environment—primarily light and darkness—and trigger physical, mental, and behavioral changes in our bodies known as circadian rhythms. These primal rhythms exert a greater influence over our weight and our health than even our metabolism and how many calories we consume.

The study of this incredibly powerful, intertwined "watch" movement is called *chronobiology*. Significant research in recent years suggests that when our circadian rhythms are disrupted by events natural and unnatural (such as overeating, lack of sleep, psychological stress, constant stimulation by technology, and drugs and chemicals in our foods), abnormalities occur in the body that lead to poor health, weight gain, and disease.

Sounds like a real bummer, no? Yup, it's true. But the good news is that what we now are beginning to understand about our circadian rhythm can help us to flip the switch, resetting our body clocks to bring our mind and body back into a healthy rhythm.

THE SUN GODDESS RULES

That big ol' ball of hot plasma at the center of the solar system is the prime energy source for all life. As Earth's rotation spins you rhythmically into dark and then light again, your body's master clock, the suprachiasmatic nucleus, inside your brain causes some pretty powerful events to happen throughout your being. Disruptions to this circadian rhythm can make it harder to fit into your favorite skinny jeans.

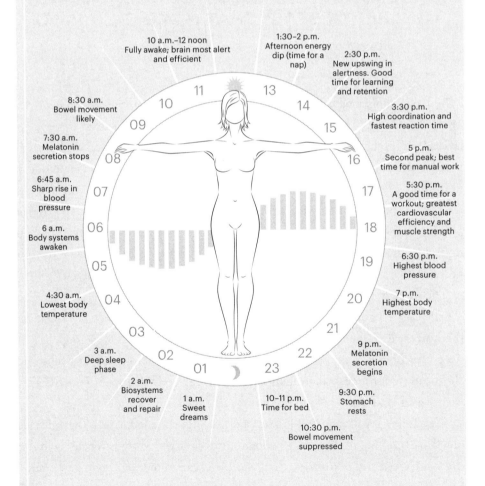

10 a.m.–12 noon
Fully awake; brain most alert and efficient

1:30–2 p.m.
Afternoon energy dip (time for a nap)

2:30 p.m.
New upswing in alertness. Good time for learning and retention

8:30 a.m.
Bowel movement likely

3:30 p.m.
High coordination and fastest reaction time

7:30 a.m.
Melatonin secretion stops

5 p.m.
Second peak; best time for manual work

6:45 a.m.
Sharp rise in blood pressure

5:30 p.m.
A good time for a workout; greatest cardiovascular efficiency and muscle strength

6 a.m.
Body systems awaken

6:30 p.m.
Highest blood pressure

4:30 a.m.
Lowest body temperature

7 p.m.
Highest body temperature

3 a.m.
Deep sleep phase

9 p.m.
Melatonin secretion begins

2 a.m.
Biosystems recover and repair

1 a.m.
Sweet dreams

10–11 p.m.
Time for bed

9:30 p.m.
Stomach rests

10:30 p.m.
Bowel movement suppressed

We've already learned that the tiny peripheral clocks all over your body are governed by a master body clock located in the hypothalamus of your brain, called the suprachiasmatic nucleus, or SCN. The SCN ultimately controls many hormones and biocycles including the feeding/eating cycle, the hunger/fullness cycle, the wake/sleep cycle, the rest-and-digest cycle, and even the rhythm to which your heart beats. In this chapter, we will explore the other biological mechanisms that influence your circadian rhythm to better understand how managing your body clock can help you to lose weight.

ATTACK OF THE ZEITGEBERS

Your circadian rhythm has been with you since the day you were born. It's built-in and self-sustaining, but that doesn't mean it doesn't change. It does!

Your body clock is adjusted by external cues called *zeitgebers,* which is a German word meaning "time giver" or "synchronizer." The most important and powerful of the zeitgebers is, you guessed it, the sun! Light entering your eyes tweaks the SCN cells and sets your circadian rhythm in motion. That's good when it follows the natural cycle of light and darkness.

But lesser zeitgebers can make your internal clock go cuckoo. Like what? Artificial light at night, processed foods, easy access to foods 24/7, mental stress and stress hormones, pharmaceutical drugs, exercise, even behavioral things such as a specific task that keeps the body alert, like following a train schedule or working the second or third shift; watching TV late at night; taking a 2-hour nap on a Saturday afternoon; or staying up all night to cram for an exam. Except for natural sunlight, all those other zeitgebers are modern-day cues that knock your clock off-kilter.

So when I say being overweight isn't your fault, I really mean it. Blame it on living in the Land of Plenty. Our Land of Plenty doesn't operate with respect to the 24-hour clock. Rather, people force themselves to work more, sleep less, and disregard the light/dark cycle. Food is available literally at the click of your computer mouse. College kids can order in pizza on their iPhones through services like Seamless, regardless of the time of day. Did you know there's a cookie company in New York City called Insomnia that offers cookies until 3 a.m.? Artificial light makes it possible for us to work 24 hours a day, 7 days a week, so we're in a constant state of alertness—another word for stress.

Think about how you feel when you travel from the East Coast of the United States

FUELING FAT

The human body is programmed to hold on to calories when it senses a food-poor environment, by slowing metabolism and increasing fat stores. When we adopt a fad diet that severely restricts calories to lose weight, our body doesn't recognize our intention for self-improvement; instead it thinks food is scarce, and it needs to switch to survival mode. So, you see, while your intention is to become healthier through dieting, you're in fact making yourself more stressed, fatter, and food obsessed.

Look at the statements below. If you identify with three or more of them, your body clock needs a reboot.

1. I have difficulty falling asleep and staying asleep.

2. I regularly travel through different time zones.

3. I find there's never enough time in the day to get house chores, work, and meal planning done.

4. I sleep less than 8 hours daily.

5. I have tried more than three diets in the past 5 years.

6. I have lost and gained back more weight when dieting.

7. I have irritable bowel syndrome or stomach/intestine issues (GI discomfort, constipation, diarrhea).

8. I consume the greatest amount of calories at night.

9. I feel constantly stressed by work and life. I have no downtime.

10. I eat in response to my stressors.

11. I do everything for everyone else but myself.

12. I hate my body.

to Europe. Your circadian rhythm is disrupted, causing jet-lag symptoms of fatigue, disorientation, and insomnia. Even when you fly from New York to Los Angeles, for example, your body clock time will be different from the time on your wristwatch.

What's amazing and at the same time dangerous is that the human body is so resilient to these disruptions, allowing you to function surprisingly well in this go-go world of 24/7 stimulation. But stop and think: Is your body functioning optimally, the way you want it to? What are the repercussions?

My client Lisa travels from NYC to London for work and returns 2 days later expecting to operate at 100 percent despite changing time zones and experiencing a different feeding/eating and light/dark cycle. Sound familiar? She then has difficulty with sleep and uses a prescription sleep aid to get back on track with her time zone. While this is a functioning body, it is clearly not an ideal situation. The body perseveres to the detriment of our body clock, our waistline, and our overall health.

Here's a more clinical example of how powerfully the body adapts to change. When you go on a calorie-restricted diet, it's fairly easy to lose weight initially. But soon the body recognizes that something's amiss. The calories aren't coming in, so it goes into preservation mode, slowing down to reduce calorie expenditure. Dr. Ralph Carson, author of *The Brain Fix,* says this is the body's innate response for survival. When the body believes it's being starved due to lack of food—rather than experiencing a mere diet to lose excess pounds gained by living in the Land of Plenty—it throttles down all physical processes. Whether it's for menstruation or metabolism, the body's preservation mode slows organ functions such as heart rate and can even cause cognitive delay. Our bodies continue to adapt to maintain life even when it's counterproductive and actually to our disadvantage.

Like Clockwork

If you wind a clock too many times and too fast, what happens? It breaks, right? Well, this happens with our body's natural processes. We run, run, run, and then we bonk out. We work, work, work, and then we have a breakdown. Our cells synchronize with our environment to function appropriately for specific times of day. However, when our clock's rhythm gets disrupted at unexpected times by food, artificial light, and stress (known as the three key disruptors), our biological pathways go haywire. This means your feeding/eating, hunger/fullness, and sleep cycles get confused and try to adapt. This can increase the risk of heart disease and even diabetes.

How the Three Key Zeitgebers
Disrupt Your Body Clock

Disruptor 1: Food

Your body clock regulates almost all hormones in your body. This is important news, especially in this day and age of insulin resistance, diabetes, polycystic ovary syndrome, and other hormone-related disorders. Here's what should happen when you eat: As food is digested, specifically carbohydrates such as fruits, beans, and breads, it enters our bloodstream as sugar. The pancreas releases the hormone insulin, which serves as a key to unlock the doorway of a cell, allowing sugar to enter your cells to create energy. What happens in between meals? The body clock is always trying to maintain a *homeostasis,* so when it senses the decrease in available sugar between meals, it releases another hormone, called *glucagon.* This natural chemical triggers your body to release the sugar stored in your muscles and liver cells, known as *glycogen,* creating blood sugar balance.

While food consumption affects the release of hormones, your hormones also follow a regular hunger/fullness cycle. The appetite hormone known as *ghrelin* is made in the stomach and relays the hunger message to the brain, telling you to find food. An easy way to remember the role of this hormone is that ghrelin sounds like *Grrr,* as in "Grrrowl, my belly is empty."

Ghrelin levels plummet after a meal, while *leptin,* the hormone responsible for indicating fullness, rises. Leptin follows the circadian rhythm—just like everything else, for that matter. For example, in the dead of night, at 2:00 a.m. when the body is supposed to be asleep, leptin peaks, rising 30 to 100 percent higher than during the morning and afternoon, when we're supposed to be active and in need of food.

These hormones are all part of the central nervous system, relaying information between the gastrointestinal tract and the brain. Besides ghrelin, the majority of the other GI hormones regulated by the body clock are satiety hormones. These chemicals all relay the message of fullness. They're secreted by the cells of the intestine as well as other parts of the body (such as the pancreas and the fat cells known as adipocytes) and are supposed to be in rhythm with the 24-hour body clock. The main ones you're probably familiar with are insulin and leptin.

Leptin is the satiety hormone. Following a meal, gastric leptin gets released directly into the GI tract, allowing you to feel full. But when the body is without adequate nutrition or has decreased body fat stores, the body clock suppresses the production of leptin. This is the body's effort to survive and adapt. When gaining weight and increasing body fat, leptin increases in accordance with an increase in your body fat mass. This means the more fat you have, the more full you feel until you develop something called *leptin resistance*.

The following chart demonstrates how certain environmental situations can affect your leptin.

	Malnutrition	Sleep deprivation	24- to 72-hour fasting	Exercise
Leptin decreases and hunger increases	X	X	X	X

	High estrogen	Insulin/carbohydrate intake	Overfeeding	High fat stores
Leptin increases and hunger decreases (except with leptin deficiency and leptin resistance)	X	X	X	X

Move Over, Insulin Resistance

Insulin is the other critical metabolic hormone. Its job is to trigger your cells to absorb sugar from the bloodstream to store and produce energy. As mentioned earlier, when the body doesn't produce enough insulin or the presence of insulin is ineffective in shuttling sugar into your cells and out of your bloodstream, prediabetes and diabetes can occur. Insulin resistance is when your body becomes insensitive to insulin.

Well, just like insulin, your body can become insensitive to the presence of leptin. As a result, the body produces more and more leptin. The body is basically signaling the need for more calories to create greater fat stores and greater production of leptin. This cycle is maladaptive in the Land of Plenty because the body programs itself to continuously eat and gain fat despite the fact that food and body fat stores are adequate. Here is another example of how eating against the clock triggers metabolic confusion and ultimately disease. Eating sugar during the dark phase (when you should be snug as a bug in bed) affects leptin. Excess simple carbohydrates knock the body clock out of rhythm, resulting in a decrease in leptin and an increase in glucose and insulin. Researchers often see leptin resistance in shift workers who eat at night and sleep during the day. They never feel full and are constantly hungry despite the fact that insulin and blood sugar are in excess. Research correlates these circumstances with obesity, significant belly fat, and metabolic syndrome.

ARE YOU A SHIFT WORKER WITHOUT A SHIFT?

If you're in a constant state of stress, never have downtime, and frequently pull all-nighters for work, your body clock can get disrupted. This is easiest to see in shift workers. Nighttime shift workers are associated with having heart disease, increased body mass, elevated blood sugar (leading to diabetes), and high cholesterol. These metabolic effects are also seen in people who function out of the normal wake/sleep cycle due to career constraints, school schedules, and social events. This could be you. Take this test to see if your lifestyle qualifies as similar to that of a shift worker.

1. Are you awake at night?

2. Do you eat when it's dark out?

3. Do you sleep more than 1 hour during daylight hours?

4. Do you have night-eating syndrome?

5. Do you skip meals all day and eat only one meal in the evening or at night?

6. Do you travel for work?

7. Do you go to sleep at a different time every night?

8. Do you wake up at a different time every morning?

9. Do you pull all-nighters?

10. Are you constantly in a state of alertness via drugs, caffeine, and/or stress?

If you answered yes to any of the above questions, hitting Reset on the body clock is a good idea!

Disruptor 2: Light

Our 24/7 lifestyle has us working in opposition to the natural rhythm of light and darkness and has triggered an epidemic of body clock disharmony. When you should be sleeping at night, you're traveling through time zones, working, and eating. When you finally try to get to sleep, your body is confused and your sleep is off.

Your body responds to light via the retina-to-brain pathway. When the light cues change to a different 24-hour light/dark cycle, the body clock adjusts. This can take days to weeks. This effort to adapt to the new light cycle deactivates the rhythm of the peripheral clocks that operate all around our bodies.

Who said humans could make their own schedules? Clearly, the body clock cannot synchronize to this modern lifestyle of jet setting and dancing till dawn. Yet we try to, and thus have paved the way to sleep disorders and sleep deprivation. The Institute of Medicine says sleep issues are so rampant, they're now a public health issue. Statistics from the Centers for Disease Control and Prevention reveal that 4 percent of Americans take prescription sleeping pills. The number is higher for women than men and does not include women taking the over-the-counter sleep hormone melatonin.

The Body Clock's Sleep Hormone

The hormone melatonin is naturally released at night to lower blood pressure and heart rate, reduce temperature, and temper cortisol to help you become sleepy. This is managed by the body clock, specifically the 24-hour rhythm and the light/dark cycle.

What happens if you challenge the body clock and don't get this release of melatonin and, as a result, don't get enough sleep? For one thing, the mechanism that makes you fat kicks in—the result of a cocktail of little insults. Lack of sleep dulls the operation of the frontal lobe, the decision-making and impulse-regulating center of your brain. A foggy frontal lobe sets you up to make poor food choices. Lack of sleep also messes with your hunger/fullness hormones ghrelin and leptin, making you prone to bingeing on calorie-dense foods. A study in the *American Journal of Clinical Nutrition* found that women who were sleep deprived tended to increase their late-night snacking, specifically on high-carbohydrate foods.

Poor-quality sleep also increases levels of the stress hormone cortisol and affects another critical metabolic hormone, insulin. University of Chicago researchers found that just 4 nights of inadequate sleep decreased total-body insulin sensitivity by an average of 16 percent and the insulin sensitivity of fat cells by 30 percent. And we know what happens when insulin becomes less effective; your body produces more and more, and elevated insulin increases body fat.

Many, many studies have demonstrated a clear association between short sleep duration with higher body weight and type 2 diabetes. Most of the research that specifically looked at the role of the body clock was done on animals and shift workers, the people who work through the night and sleep during the daylight to enable our 24/7 lifestyle.

Now, for a minute, just think about how awful your body feels when you pull an all-nighter. Do you have any friends who work through the night at a bar or in a factory? Do they ever adjust to this schedule? Do they ever complain of weight and/or

GUT CHECK
How Your "Second Brain" Affects Your Body Clock and Weight

Your brain and belly are like very tight sisters who can finish each other's sentences or who know instinctively when the other is upset. They are clearly connected.

Have you ever experienced a "gut feeling" when interviewing for a job? When faced with an important decision, have you ever had to just "go with your gut instinct"? It's not just metaphorical; the physical connection between the gut and the mind can indeed have a profound effect on our mood, our weight, and our health.

In 1996, Dr. Michael Gershon, chairman of the department of anatomy and cell biology at Columbia University, brilliantly recognized the gastrointestinal tract as "the second brain." He wrote a book about it called *The Second Brain*, in which he explained that the brain and belly communicate along what's known as the brain-gut axis via the vagus nerve. The second brain is lined with neuropeptides and receptors that are largely responsible for mood and therefore have a lot to do with the food we consume. No wonder, then, that if you're angry with yourself or a friend, this emotional stomach issues? I can tell you right now, their minds and bodies never feel right. Perhaps you've seen your hospital nurse or doctor with red eyes as she comes off the night shift. Do these people ever adjust? No, they don't. Many of my clients work these hours and are fraught with all types of GI symptoms and complaints. They say they never know when to eat, they never are able to sleep, and, well, they just can't lose weight.

It's not logical nor does it feel normal to humans to operate against the body clock. We were designed to sleep when it's dark and consume the majority of our nutrition during the daylight waking hours. Research has shown that shift workers, individuals with nighttime eating routines, and rodents in studies who are fed during the dark periods significantly increase their body mass. That kind of shift-worker-like lifestyle also puts you at a 40 percent increased risk for cardiovascular disease compared with someone who follows the light/darkness rhythm set by the sun.

(continued on page 32)

upset can cause stomach upset or even trigger emotional eating.

The mind-gut connection flows the other way too. Research shows that the trillions of microbes residing in the gut respond directly to emotional stress. A bacterial imbalance in the gut due to stress, or a body clock that's not in rhythm, may cause anxiety and depressive-like behaviors, according to researchers studying animals at McMaster University. The same mechanism can trigger inflammatory disorders such as arthritis, nonalcoholic fatty liver disease, and weight gain.

But there's evidence that improving the balance of gut bacteria through diet can be the answer to nudging the two brains back into a healthy rhythm. In one study UCLA researchers found that women who regularly ate probiotics, beneficial bacteria, through yogurt showed improvements in brain function. Other research published in the British Journal of Nutrition suggests that consuming probiotics could help people lose weight. The researchers believe that the probiotics helped subjects drop weight by making their intestinal walls less permeable to molecules linked to obesity.

CLOCK TALK
The Terminology of What Makes You Tick

Autonomic nervous system: The overall system that regulates heart rate, digestion, respiratory rate, pupil response, urination, and sexual arousal largely unconsciously. It controls the stress response, known as the fight-or-flight response, by way of the following two systems.

Sympathetic nervous system: The part of the autonomic system responsible for activating the physiological changes that occur during the fight-or-flight response by releasing norepinephrine.

Parasympathetic nervous system: The part of the autonomic system that activates the "rest-and-digest" cycle by causing the release of the neurotransmitter acetylcholine; this system counters the sympathetic system after a fight-or-flight response.

Cell-autonomous circadian clock: The system that allows the body's cells to anticipate a repeated daily trigger before it actually occurs. There are the following two types of circadian clocks.

Enteral circadian clock: The part of the suprachiasmatic nucleus that manages feeding, sleeping, waking, learning, memorizing, and glucose metabolism/insulin secretion on a cellular level.

Peripheral circadian clock: The part of the central nervous system located in the body tissues.

Circadian rhythm: The body clock rhythm closely synchronized to a 24-hour period.

Cortisol: The stress hormone produced by the adrenal glands that follows a 24-hour rhythm with the highest level within the first hour of waking (known as cortisol-awakening response or CAR), a dip between 3 and 4 p.m., and the lowest level in the evening.

Cortisol-awakening response (CAR): The trigger for an increase in cortisol that occurs within the first 30 to 60 minutes of waking.

Diurnal rhythm: The body rhythm synchronized with the day/night, light/
dark cycle.

Entrainment: An adaption/response over time to an imposed cue such
as artificial light or food.

Fight, flight, or freeze response: The body's stress response releasing
epinephrine and cortisol from the adrenal glands to increase blood
pressure and blood sugar and boost energy by utilizing the sugar and
fatty acids; this response also slows or stops the action of the stomach
and upper intestine. Most people know this as the fight-or-flight
response.

Metabolic syndrome: A condition of insulin resistance, high triglycerides, high low-density lipoprotein (LDL) cholesterol, high fasting
glucose, and abdominal obesity largely seen in overweight people and
in normal-weight people with large weight fluctuations from yo-yo
dieting.

Rest-and-digest response: During this response governed by the parasympathetic system, the body activates the release of the neurotransmitter acetylcholine and returns to a state of balance following the
stress response known as fight, flight, or freeze.

Zeitgeber: A cue (such as light or food) that synchronizes the circadian
clock.

Disruptor 3: Stress

Some stress is good. Positive stress is the excitement we feel when we're ready to walk down the aisle, dressed and beautiful on our wedding day, or the thrill of the challenge we face in completing a mud run with our friends. At the opposite side of the spectrum is negative stress. It's the daily stress we feel when juggling our responsibilities, dealing with an angry friend, or worrying about paying our bills. Don't forget about the constant negative food and body thoughts, plus the self-conscious thoughts you have while walking poolside in your bathing suit. This is the intense, around-the-clock stress of almost every woman.

The body clock's response to the above stressors is to flood the body with the infamous hormone cortisol. This hormone affects almost every organ and tissue. Its main job is to help your body prepare for fight or flight in response to stress by regulating blood pressure, heart function, and kidney function. It also slows the body's immune response and regulates metabolism.

The hypothalamus in your brain triggers the pituitary to signal the adrenal glands to produce cortisol. When cortisol is produced, its presence signals back to the pituitary gland and hypothalamus to stop releasing cortisol. This is called a feedback loop, and it's one of the functions of the 24-hour body clock.

For example, you're driving in the country with the top down, singing your favorite song, when a deer shoots across the road. You automatically stop singing, grip the wheel, and slam on the brakes. You have just triggered a healthy stress response, the way your body was designed to function. When you come to a stop, you realize no one is hurt, not even the deer. Your palms are sweaty and your heart is beating faster. You try to calm your heart rate. The cortisol that surged when you hit the brakes now sends the message that it's no longer needed. This is the feedback loop. Eventually you return to a relaxed state: homeostasis.

All would be idyllic if our bodies truly functioned this way. Unfortunately, the negative stress caused by the modern age can basically put your body's system into the fight, flight, or freeze mode, 24 hours a day, 7 days a week. This means your body is constantly in overdrive. Your adrenal glands are pumping cortisol. The glands are supposed to signal the release of cortisol and then back off. However, in chronic perceived stress, the cortisol feedback system gets disrupted, and your stressed body no longer backs off. You're constantly on edge, putting your fists up, ready for the fight, and your body clock is overwound and out of whack.

Here's how a constant flood of cortisol affects your weight. In a stressed state, your blood sugar is continually elevated, triggering the need for insulin and over-stimulating the pancreas. The constant elevation of cortisol, blood sugar, and insulin increases your appetite and negatively affects your body weight. What's more, excess cortisol and insulin tend to cause the body to deposit fat in the abdominal area and around important organs, where it secretes damaging chemicals.

A Combo Deal

The three key zeitgebers—food, light, and stress—are difficult to avoid in the 24/7 Land of Plenty. Consider this scenario: You just moved to a new city, started working at a new company, and are working 15-hour days. You have yet to make friends, because you're constantly working. You can't sleep. You order meals at your desk and feel a bit homesick. Things do improve, but with friends and a fast-paced career, you never have downtime. You race to the gym at 5:00 a.m. to squeeze in a workout, skip breakfast to keep calories down, and function on Diet Cokes all day. You're promoted and given more responsibility and are now beyond stressed. This is your life, and there's no stopping.

You're even more upset when you visit the doctor to learn you've gained weight and increased your blood pressure. Just last month you did the 7-day juice cleanse. You despise your failure with the scale. Why is it that your body can't lose weight? Then your doctor reports back that your blood work indicates extremely high cortisol levels. You think about how stressed you feel, how tense your muscles are, how quickly you get irritated, or how easily you cry. Your adrenal glands are now working against you.

This is an example of our modern-day stress. Can you see any parts of your life in the composite above? My guess is you can. Our modern world affects all our body clocks to some degree. When our master clock becomes desynchronized by poor food choices, overeating and/or eating at the wrong times, lack of sleep, and chronic stress, we feel ill, we gain weight, and we reach for high-calorie foods to soothe our discomfort. This is not healthy living. This is the kind of lifestyle situation that adds pounds to our bodies. You know the phrase "three strikes and you're out"? Well, our diets, sleep habits, and stress have struck our body clock. And it's time to reset it before the seventh-inning stretch.

Part II

RESET YOUR BODY CLOCK

CHAPTER
4

Reset Button #1: Change Your Food 'Tude

MASTER THE PILLARS OF POSITIVE NUTRITION AND LEARN TO RECOGNIZE REAL HUNGER

C hanging your attitude toward food is the first of three reset buttons that will reboot your master body clock back into rhythm. The other two effective resets involve reestablishing healthy patterns of eating and sleeping. You will find those resets in Chapters 5 and 6, respectively. But we start here with your mind, because it's your most powerful instrument of change.

Healthy eating is about eating mindfully, that is, thinking about your internal body cues such as hunger and fullness, not just chowing down willy-nilly. It's also about being cognizant of time, because when you eat can have as much effect on your body clock as what you eat and how much. It's making a decision to have a certain food or combination of foods while knowing how they will affect your mood and energy level. Here's a real-world example of eating mindfully: You choose to eat a slice of decadent chocolate cake during the day, following a high-protein meal, rather than eating the cake as a bedtime snack because you know the protein meal will counter the sugar surge from the cake, and the daytime hit of caffeine from the chocolate will likely wear off before bedtime. You see, foods are powerful zeitgebers and can throw a monkey wrench into your body clock's plans to handle sugar properly and shut down for the night.

The physical clock disrupters—a quarter pound of sugar and flour in your gut and caffeine in your bloodstream—are easy to recognize. But there's a more insidious influencer affecting your body clock that you might not be aware of: your food 'tude. The good versus evil, eat this, not that approach to food selection puts a negative spin on what should be a positive experience.

By learning to recognize the type of hunger you're feeling whenever the pangs bang and practicing the Five Pillars of Positive Nutrition, you'll develop a healthier attitude toward hunger that aligns naturally with your biorhythms. Let's start with the tools you need to accomplish that.

THE FIVE PILLARS OF POSITIVE NUTRITION
1. Adopt an "All Foods Fit" Philosophy

All foods provide nutrition but in different amounts based on nutrient composition and quantity consumed. Adopting this "everything is A-okay" attitude will automatically help you learn to eat all foods in moderation and prevent you from feeling deprived and restricted from eating foods that happen to have made some magazine's "do not eat" list. Of course, All Foods Fit is not a green light to eat all foods, all the time, in any amount. That would be silly. Let me make the point this way: One meal or even one week without fresh vegetables will not affect your metabolism and body clock, but one week of restricting your calories or eating extra-large calzones and pints of Cherry Garcia certainly will.

The All Foods Fit philosophy is your escape from the dieting roller coaster. And it's an awesome way to avoid the confusing information about food and diet that's making your head spin. Food science is constantly contradicting itself. First we're told to eat carbs, and then we're told to avoid carbs at all costs. We were also told that fat was bad, but then we learned that fats such as olive oil, avocado, and other monounsaturated fats were needed for good health. I mean, of course we need fat in our diet. We especially need omega-3 fatty acids, since our bodies cannot make these essential fatty acids. That's why they're called "essential"! We learned too much vitamin A may cause cancer. Well, anything in excess can become unhealthy. Even attempting to be too thin or too healthy becomes harmful. So science is really telling us to be moderate: Eat lots of different foods in moderation and be mindful of the types of foods that keep you satiated and those that drive up your blood sugar. All Foods Fit means "no crazy restrictions on deliciousness" as long as you're eating mindfully.

2. Use Neutral Food Language

Sorry, I don't like the latest pop diet phrase: Eat clean. I understand the prescription to encourage folks to choose fresh foods over processed ones. But you see it's that same ol' good versus evil, eat this, not that approach to nutrition that can lead to body clock disruption. Think about it: What's the opposite of a clean food? A dirty one? A McIntosh apple that slipped out of your hand into the mud? By adopting neutral food language, you eliminate the judgments that can fuel guilt and become a real Debbie Downer at a dinner party. So out with the food labeling. Ben and Jerry aren't bad guys. Eating kale won't get you into heaven, but if you eat too much, your skin may turn orange. I've heard people call carbohydrates the devil incarnate, yet apples, sweet potatoes, beans, and quinoa are carbs, and they're pretty darn healthy to eat. Let's make a deal: Foods aren't good or bad. They're just food.

3. Be an Honorable Eater

Often a client will visit me and say she had a bad day and feels guilty because she had some chips at lunchtime or Dunkin' Munchkins with her coffee at a friend's place. "I was bad today," clients will often say, or "I ate an Oreo." Or "Ugh, I ate through all my points before noon, so I just gave up and ate my way through the rest of the day. What a loser. I've got no discipline!"

Errrr. Do you hear me slamming on your brakes? Stop what you're doing! Change your focus from counting calories, using points, or using a body scale as a way to determine your worth as a human being. Instead let the thought of "valuing and honoring your body" help you establish healthy eating habits. It may sound something like this: "Today I listened to my body—I ate when I was hungry and stopped when I was full. I ate a kale-tofu salad for lunch and had cookies with milk for a side. What a great day!"

4. Don't Treat Yourself Like a Dog

Say it with me: Dogs get treats, humans eat snacks. That's right—going forward, I want you to stop thinking of tasty tidbits of food as a reward or treat for "good" behavior. Food is food. It is eaten for fuel and other reasons, but we don't place certain food types on a pedestal to be worshiped as special and craved. This mentality is likely to cause you to overeat this "treat" and wreak havoc on your body clock. Instead treat yourself to vacations, flowers, and new lipsticks as rewards for your accomplishments. But keep food out of it.

5. Love Fat; It's Not Your Foe

Whether it's fat on your body or in your food, stop judging it. It's not bad or ugly or evil. In either place, food or body, it's natural, healthy, and needed. Fat in your food is an essential macronutrient. You can have fat on your body and be beautiful. Whatever names you were called as a child, whatever comments people make about your body, just know we all are imperfect in our own ways. The Body Clock Diet is about balance with your biological systems. If you're trying to attain the perfection you see in the Photoshopped pictures of models in magazines, you will set yourself up for a broken body clock. So let's neutralize the negativity surrounding the word *fat* to help our society redefine beauty and overall health. You can be healthy with fat on your body. You can also be unhealthy with fat on your body. Don't judge a book just by its cover.

ID YOUR HUNGER TYPE

Read the Five Pillars of Positive Nutrition over and over again. Read them before bed and before you leave the house in the morning. Take a picture of the pillars and keep the photo stored on your phone. They are your new mantra for balancing your clock.

Now, there's another powerful cognitive tool that will help you reset your body clock: being a mindful eater—that is, being able to identify the type of hunger you're feeling so you're better able to generate a healthy response that keeps your circadian clock in rhythm.

Let's define each of the four types of hunger: emotional, behavioral, physical, and hedonic.

Emotional Hunger

We all flock to food as a way to celebrate or to make us feel better or even numb in times of emotional stress. Emotional eating can happen because you're happy and you want to celebrate. Perhaps you were promoted at work and feel you deserve a dinner celebration. What about graduating from college? You celebrate with dinner and drinks. There may be a sense of entitlement with emotional eating.

Emotional hunger can also occur when we feel sad, disappointed, alone, empty, or even angry. It can be the act of eating to punish yourself rather than to comfort you. Some of my clients eat as a form of self-sabotage. They share with me: "It's to punish myself, as I don't deserve to be happy; I don't want to feel attractive." More than one of my clients have shared that they eat to prevent weight loss or more

LEAVE SOME COOKIES ON THE PLATE

One of my favorite definitions of *normal eating* was eloquently described by registered dietitian and licensed clinical social worker Ellyn Satter. She spoke of sometimes eating too much, sometimes too little, and sometimes just the right amount. She also included "being able to leave some cookies on the plate." I love her definition and encourage you to look it up. I'm not sure that the label *normal* applies. Frankly, in this modern world, I don't know that there is such a thing as normal eating, since the norm seems to be dieting or disordered eating. Perhaps *balanced eating* is a better phrase? Or *honor eating*? We'll call it *mindful eating*. It's about recognizing your physical and emotional needs for food and choosing an empowering path.

specifically to prevent expectations. They tell me they believe the additional weight will lessen expectations from their parents or even their boss, saying "This prevents disappointing others or having to live up to higher expectations." Some women believe they're unworthy of feeling proud, attractive, or intelligent.

And then some of you may identify with my other clients, who eat to punish themselves for not having eaten perfectly during the week or, once again, not having lost weight after "dieting all week." Is this you? Let it marinate. Be mindful of why you eat and if the hunger you're fueling is something other than a true physical reaction signaling the need for nutritional energy. Biological factors can also trigger emotional hunger and eating. Consider those ever-fluctuating female hormones.

But hormones aren't entirely to blame. Emotional eating may also be a way to avoid dealing with psychological stress. Eating away our feelings can be a more comfortable, safer way to deal with them than confronting a problem head-on.

Emotional Hunger	Physical Hunger
Comes on suddenly	Comes on gradually
Craves comfort foods	Is satisfied by all foods
Isn't satisfied with a full belly	Stops when you're full
Triggers feelings of guilt and lack of control	Sends the belly-brain sensations of fullness through hormones

Erase Emotional Eating

If you recognize that you've been eating for emotional reasons, we're going to remedy this situation from the inside out and the outside in. We'll provide you with a meal structure in each phase of the Body Clock Diet. This is the "outside-in" approach and is meant to be temporary. This will help to restore the natural biological rhythm you were born with.

Now, to change your relationship with food-mind-body, you will need to develop coping skills and adaptions. Rereading the Five Pillars of Positive Nutrition can help. Here's another of my favorites: using a comfort card.

Comfort Card

Grab an index card. Think about the top five most effective coping skills you know to minimize your feelings of stress and anxiety. Ideas for coping skills may include yogic breathing, journaling, drawing, painting, coloring, sculpting, playing music, crying, talking to a friend, and so on. Healthy non-self-destructive distractions could be playing solitaire, knitting, going for a walk, scrapbooking, collaging, or doing a crossword puzzle. The idea is to find ways to change automatic behavior to a mindful choice and try distracting yourself to break the cycle of reaching for food as a salve to soothe the emotions.

It's similar to the scenario we learned about in science class—you know, the one about Pavlov's dog. Pavlov conditioned his dog so that every time Pavlov rang a bell, the dog came running. He came running because he knew food would be waiting. Soon Pavlov took the dog food out of the scenario. The dog continued to go to Pavlov when he rang the bell. He was now conditioned to go to his owner. Well, we need to condition you similarly. Instead of being conditioned to comfort yourself with food, you need to employ one or more of the skills and/or distractions on your comfort card until it becomes your automatic thought and/or action. We call it a comfort card because it needs to be something you enjoy. If not, there's no way you'll pass up food for the idea of doing something unfulfilling.

My clients love knitting, yoga, and art projects. Michaels craft stores get a lot of business from them. By the way, there are very cool adult coloring books called *Enchanted Forest* and *Secret Garden* by the artist Johanna Basford. My clients use the books to help calm and distract themselves from eating for nonphysical reasons. Another artist, Angie Grace, creates beautiful black-and-white coloring pages meant to melt stress away.

Create your own comfort card or use the sample card on the next page when you start Phase 1. We show an example card filled out by one of my clients to give you an idea of what yours may look like.

You don't have to wait for Chapter 7. Start using your personal coping skills and distractions right now.

Every time you eat, take a mindful breath (any deep breath will suffice) and identify what type of hunger you're responding to. Is it emotional, behavioral, or physical? If it's emotional or behavioral, grab your card and work your way down your list as needed.

SAMPLE COMFORT CARD	
*Always begin by repeating the Five Pillars of Positive Nutrition	
1.	Journal what I'm feeling in my new diary
2.	Paint a picture
3.	Play the piano
4.	Go for a walk with my best friend
5.	Knit for 10 minutes or longer
6.	Work on my arts and crafts project

MY COMFORT CARD	
*Always begin by repeating the Five Pillars of Positive Nutrition	
1.	
2.	
3.	
4.	
5.	
6.	

Behavioral Hunger

Behavioral hunger is the act of eating out of habit or to pass time. It's something to do. An example of behavioral hunger and eating is going to Starbucks for a Frappuccino every summer afternoon just because it's hot out and, well, it's simply what you do when the clock strikes 3:00 every day. Another example is going to lunch at 1:30 with the girls from the office because you want to be part of the group and don't want to miss the social fun even if you already ate at your desk at noon because you were starving.

Behavioral eating is programmed into us when we go to school and are forced to eat lunch at 10:30 a.m. despite having eaten breakfast at 9:00 a.m. Every time you come home, you automatically walk straight into the kitchen and eat despite the time of day or night. It is your habit. It is your norm. You don't even think about it. You just do it.

Moms: Are you teaching your children behavioral eating? You are if you encourage them to clean their plate even if they feel full and aren't hungry any longer. Were you taught this? How many of you still struggle with the learned behavior of the "clean-your-plate club"? You go to a restaurant where they serve a portion twice as large as your normal dinner and you finish the entire portion. You eat the entire double-size entrée because you're programmed to clean the plate. You're robotic about feeding and eating. And let's not forget what we were taught as little tots. A birthday means pizza, soda, and birthday cake. You get it? This is learned behavior. It's almost like the "see-food diet"—you see food and are behaviorally conditioned to eat it.

Boot Behavioral Eating

Simply identifying yourself as a behavioral eater is a positive and truly awakening step. This is the start of mastering mindfulness. Observing or being aware of your thoughts, feelings, and actions is mindfulness. A few pointers can help you become more aware of when you're eating for behavioral reasons.

1. Sit at a table when you eat any type of food. This means no eating while walking, driving, or standing.

2. Eat with humans, not technology. Say goodbye to iPads, PC screens, and television screens. This translates to no popcorn at the movies. This is such a commonly

taught form of behavioral eating. You grow up learning *I eat candy and popcorn at the movie theater and hot dogs with cotton candy at the baseball game.* What ever happened to eating for physical hunger before, during, or after the event?

3. Embrace boredom when you eat. Clients tell me it's so boring to eat without the TV on or other distractions to occupy their minds. Yup, that's the point. Distractions keep you from focusing on your food and your satiety. Get rid of them. Enjoy eating and knowing when to stop.

4. Log feelings, thoughts, and actions before you even take that first bite. Now you have to make the decision to eat or not to eat. This is not a game, so there is no cheating. Just decide.

5. Dial your belly-brain phone line. Ask yourself if you're physically hungry. Think when was the last time you ate. Could you be eating as an activity? A social event? A distraction? A procrastination? All that is—you got it—behavioral eating.

6. Break the habit by using the comfort card. Just do something else!

Now you know how to handle both emotional and behavioral hungers. The next hunger is the belly-brain dialogue.

Physical Hunger

This type of hunger is the golden cue! This is belly-brain communication signaling the need for fuel. Physical hunger is the mind-body's response to an empty stomach, low blood sugar, and/or decreased fat stores. Physical hunger is your body's prompt to try to return to homeostasis. It's the need for additional calories to continue living—breathing, keeping your heart beating, walking, and talking—as well as to maintain the body's underlying circuitry such as the immune response or sending oxygen to the muscles. All these processes require calories. It's the real deal, the legit reason to feed oneself.

Do you really know what it feels like to be hungry? If not, don't worry. The Body Clock Meal Structure reset in Chapter 5 will help your hunger and fullness cues to return.

Tastes So Good! Hedonic Hunger

There's another type of hunger to be aware of—hedonic hunger—and it's driven by the sheer enjoyment of eating a food because it's highly tasty and decreases stress temporarily. You don't need the calories, but you eat them not out of habit or to relieve stress, but simply because the food tastes soooooo good! I'm thinking of cupcakes right now. How about you? Or barbecue potato chips; remember those? Hedonic hunger is the body's reaction to yummy food everywhere and all the time. It's thinking and obsessing about the food much like someone addicted to gambling or even drugs would.

In fact, highly palatable foods can seem as addictive as alcohol because they activate a reward system in the brain that motivates us to seek them out over and over. Food manufacturers, especially those who make processed snacks, engineer foods to have a higher reward value by combining fat, starch, sugar, salt, and glutamate in a mix that simply won't let you stop at just one.

It's no wonder hedonic hunger is closely correlated with an increase in body weight. Hedonic eating may trigger leptin resistance, where it's difficult to feel full and satisfied, so you keep on eating. For example, a 2012 study conducted at the Monell Chemical Senses Research Center found that obese women took longer

Six Hunger Hints

Listen inward for these hints of physical hunger.

1. Both your brain and your second brain (your belly) send a message that you need to eat.

2. You feel slightly weakened; you may even feel shaky.

3. You feel mentally foggy; it's harder to focus.

4. You have a sensation of emptiness in your belly area.

5. You become slightly irritated and emotional.

6. You just know—it's a gut feeling.

than lean women did to get accustomed to a sweet solution, suggesting that this could delay satiation, increase meal time, and result in overeating.

My client Aubrey, who shares her story in this book, often reported hedonic hunger. Just walking to my office was an obstacle course because there's a food venue almost every 30 feet along 14th Street in New York City. The smells of the food would be so difficult to resist. Plus, she was thinking about food 24/7, even if it wasn't present. If you can't sympathize with Aubrey, imagine you're a child. Mom tells you she is making a batch of your favorite cookies after school. You're salivating at the idea of this favorite cookie as you walk home that day. Upon entering the house, you smell the sweetness and feel the warmth. You imagine the chocolate melting on your hands and in your mouth. Screech. The music stops. Mom serves them to your brother's friends, not you. That's how it feels to have hedonic hunger. The hard reality is that the food doesn't even need to be present to give you these thoughts. The memory of that food or the smell is strong enough.

Be aware of hedonic hunger and make sure you differentiate it from other types of hunger. And know the foods that can trigger it. Remember, all foods can fit.

When a watch breaks, we take it to the repair store or get a new battery. Our batteries have a long life. Your body clock needs simply to be reset. Eating in accordance with the simple meal structure we provide in Phase 1 will help to reconnect you with your body clock while teaching you how to use the body clock's rhythm to your advantage. You only need to identify which of the three main hungers you're experiencing and start implementing the comfort card and strategies for booting behavioral eating. Two weeks later, you'll be in the perfect position to dive into the cues of the hunger/fullness cycle.

As you turn to Chapter 5, know that the meal structure you're about to incorporate daily will lead you to create a new healthy habit of mindful eating.

CHAPTER
5

Reset Button #2: Eat, Snack, Eat, Snack, Eat

FALL INTO THE DRUMBEAT OF AN EATING STRUCTURE TO SYNCHRONIZE YOUR CLOCKS AND DEFEAT TEMPTATION

Be careful out there, ladies. Dietary destruction lurks around every corner. Holiday parties with tables upon tables piled high with so much deliciousness someone jokes, "That could feed a small country!" Big bowls of leftover Halloween candy on the kitchen counter that you just can't waste. The box of birthday doughnuts left in the coffee room for all to share. Enormous mounds of pasta at your favorite Italian restaurant and cannoli sweetly calling your name from the dessert cart.

Food. It's everywhere you look. And, as I mentioned before, most of us practice the see-food diet: When we see food, we eat it.

Our access to inexpensive, abundant food is a blessing, for sure, but one that's messing up our body clocks and making it harder to squeeze into our fave jeans. As we have learned, our circadian rhythm is *entrained,* or synchronized, by environmental cues called *zeitgebers*. The most powerful zeitgeber is light; its influence on your main clock is well documented. The second, less-understood cue is food or the lack of food (feeding/fasting), which affects the peripheral clocks in every cell of the body.

Having food always within reach—or a few phone clicks away to be delivered to you—can nudge your circadian rhythm out of alignment. Cutting calories or skipping meals can do it too. For example, in the morning, your main body clock responds to light from the sun (rise and shine; it's time to start the day). But if you skip breakfast, your peripheral clocks get a different message (we're staying in bed). That contradiction puts your clocks out of sync with one another. Researchers at the Yale School of Medicine, in a 3-year study on lab mice, found that when mice ate at key times of the day, which varied depending on sleep schedule, their bodies function at their best. That's the goal of the Body Clock Diet Reset Button #2—to use the power of meal structure to reset and rev up your metabolism and to override cravings that derail weight loss.

MEAL STRUCTURE TO THE RESCUE

The Body Clock Diet meal structure prevents you from engaging in emotional, behavioral, or hedonic eating by structuring your meal times, amounts, and even combinations of food. Phase 1 of this program is designed to be more prescriptive

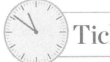 Ticktock Tip

Are You Hungry or Hangry?

Even anger can send you to the pantry for a fix of something sweet. Next time you can't determine if a craving is a real hunger pang or the result of emotional or behavioral hunger, ask yourself this question: If a big garden salad with grilled, sliced chicken breast was ready for you on the kitchen table, would you be hungry enough to eat it? If that appeals to you, you're physically hungry. If it doesn't and you still feel like hunting for a bag of chips, try to distract yourself with tips from "Boot Behavioral Eating" on page 45 or whip out your comfort card to stifle the craving.

and strict than the other two. I liken it to playing T-ball as a kid. (I have T-ball on the brain because of my own kids.) In T-ball, a kid is given a small baseball bat, a softer ball, and a T-stand to hold the ball stationary while he swings at it. Once a kid masters smacking a ball into the outfield from a T-stand, the coaches take the stand away and start pitching to the kid. The player gains more freedom and is ready to face greater challenges with his newly developed skills.

This is what you'll do during the first 2 weeks of the Body Clock Diet—get into the swing of eating at regular intervals, which will establish the basic skills to advance to less structure, and thus more freedom, where mindful eating will be your powerful guide.

Principles of Meal Structure

In Phase 1, you'll be eating small meals every 2 to 3 hours—three main meals and two snacks. Why? For one thing, it helps teach your mind and body that food is never very far away. It's always coming shortly, so don't get anxious. This behavioral training helps to prevent overeating or bingeing. Eating every 2 to 3 hours also prepares you for the release of ghrelin, the hormone that controls hunger and drives appetite. Ghrelin typically spikes after about 3 hours of fasting or if the body feels deprived of carbs, so eating with regularity helps tame the hunger trigger.

In Phase 1, you'll learn to eat when your stress hormone cortisol is low and your "I'm satisfied" hormone leptin is high. You will eat lunch earlier in the day and learn when to use skills to overcome behavioral eating at night. This structured eating will eliminate eating for hedonic hunger and leptin resistance.

As you progress through Phases 2 and 3, the time between meals and snacks will increase to an average of 3 to 4 hours. This is consistent with the rate at which your stomach empties, your blood sugar lowers, and a refuel becomes necessary.

To synchronize with your clock, it's important to keep blood sugar levels stable and avoid dramatic spikes in insulin. You can achieve this by eating what I call mixed meals, which contain all three macronutrients: carbohydrates, proteins, and fats. Don't worry; the combo will keep you energized as well as full and satisfied between meals. It's a simple-to-follow rule that will also help you to prevent metabolic disorders like prediabetes, diabetes, and the cornucopia of disorders surrounding heart disease. Here's a sample of common foods that fit into the three macronutrient groups.

Carbohydrates

Breads	Fruits	Beans and legumes
Pasta	Vegetables, especially starchy ones like potatoes	Rice
Cookies, cakes, pastries		Low-fat dairy
		Sugar*

*For a list of synonyms for sugar, see "Hide 'n' Sweet" on the next page.

Proteins

Eggs	Pork	Beans
Poultry	Lamb	Nuts and nut butters
Seafood	Yogurt	Cheeses
Beef	Tofu	

Fats

Avocado	Canola oil	Whole-fat milk
Olives	Nuts and nut butters	Cheeses
Olive oil	Butter	Cookies, cakes, pastries

Another important aspect of the meal structure is that it provides adequate calories to prevent excessive slowing of the metabolism, also known as maladaptive thermogenesis.

Principles of the Women's Health Body Clock Meal Structure

1. Meals are timed on average every 3 hours.

2. Timed meals are consistent with the 24-hour body clock.

3. Mixed meals contain all three macronutrients.

4. The majority of meals are homemade with more whole foods than processed foods.

5. Warm water in the morning helps stimulate gastric motility. (Coffee is off-limits until later.)

Time of Day—Meal Structure Management

Our body clock sets insulin to be the highest in the early morning hours. Because our insulin is already high in the a.m., it's best to eat a mixed meal (containing carbohydrates, proteins, and fats) with a moderate amount of carbohydrates to prevent the insulin from increasing further and contributing to greater insulin resistance and abdominal obesity. As mentioned earlier, it's important to eat an adequate breakfast and not skip it to keep your various body clocks in harmony. And studies do show that breaking the nighttime fast is an effective technique for revving a sluggish morning metabolism and ultimately losing weight. A study in a recent issue of the journal *Obesity* found that women who ate their largest meal at breakfast and their smallest for dinner shed more than twice as much weight over 12 weeks as those whose meal sizes were reversed.

Another important element of this meal structure is the timing of lunch. Current research in the *International Journal of Obesity* studied 420 subjects in Spain over 20 weeks while they followed a Mediterranean diet. Despite eating the same amount of nutrients, the subjects who ate lunch earlier experienced faster and greater weight loss. The study noted that the individuals who tended to be night owls (with a tendency to function better later in the day) were more likely to be late

Hide 'n' Sweet

Scan a product's ingredients list for these aliases for sugar:

Agave	Fructose	Maltodextrin
Barley malt	Fruit juice	Maple syrup
Brown rice syrup	Juice concentrate	Molasses
Corn syrup	High-fructose corn syrup	Organic cane juice
Dextrose		Sorghum
Evaporated cane juice	Honey	Sucrose
	Lactose	Turbinado

eaters, while the early "lunchers" were more likely to be "rise and shine" people and didn't skip breakfast. Finally, the meal structure also provides a meal to counter the midafternoon cortisol crash that is a function of the body clock. See "Time to Tune the Cortisol Clock" for Tame Temptation Tools to implement as part of your meal structure management.

TIME TO TUNE THE CORTISOL CLOCK

That 3-to-4 p.m., can't-keep-your-eyes-open time of day is sometimes worse than getting out of your warm, cozy bed. Our blood sugar crashes post-lunch, and before long, our eyelids are just too heavy to stay open. This occurs because our cortisol falls at this time of day. (It may start to fall as early as 2 p.m.) We become less alert, and our work can suffer. You want candy or a sugar rush to reverse this awful feeling.

In high school and even college, I experienced this lull at midday every day. Now I notice this happening to me at work only when my sleep pattern is off. Then I run out for an afternoon coffee in between clients to oppose this body clock mechanism. Can you relate? Well, this is the time to turn on all the lights and move! Read the Tame Temptation Tools below to reset your midafternoon glucose/cortisol crash.

Tame Temptation Tools

1. Eat moderate carbs with protein and fat at lunch to prevent a blood sugar roller coaster that ends in an energy slump in the early afternoon.

2. When you feel the sleepiness coming on, stand up, do a wall stretch, or strike a yoga pose, such as Warrior 1.

3. Ride it out with a power nap (10 minutes will do it—no excuses, ladies!).

4. Throw on your favorite high-energy tunes.

5. Walk it off (10 minutes combats the sleep battle).

6. Feel free to caffeinate (as long as it doesn't affect your sleep cycle).

Trick or Treat:
A Broken Clock Can Get You to Eat Too Much

The meal structure is necessary when trying to reset your body clock and lose weight. It serves to counter the leptin resistance that was discussed in Chapter 3. Leptin resistance and the false hunger known as hedonic hunger come under the umbrella of physical hunger (remember the different types of hunger from Chapter 4). But with both hedonic hunger and leptin resistance, you're eating for what feels like, but isn't, a biological need for food. Your body clock may be desynchronized from diet-induced obesity (very low-calorie fad diets can cause your metabolism to decrease). When this happens, you can't go straight to using hunger/fullness cues to regulate your eating, because your body is working against you. You feel hungry, never get full, and gain more weight. Using the Phase 1 meal structure eliminates the guessing game and gives you the opportunity to reset your feedback system. If you are truly leptin resistant or deficient, the meals are portioned so you will never have to worry about how much to eat. They're also balanced with the necessary macronutrients to manage leptin, insulin, and glucose. By eating satiating foods, you will learn to conquer hedonic eating by feeling satisfied.

The *Women's Health* Body Clock Diet recognizes that physical hunger is the golden cue to satisfy the biological need for food. We know that this system is related to the circadian rhythm and the second brain, and that sometimes your physical hunger for food isn't truly a physical need. To effectively reset the body clock, one must start to overcome restrained eating and get on a schedule of regular fueling, which we nutritionists call an external eating style. As you progress toward mindful eating practices, it will help to understand the terms *restrained eater* and *external eating*.

A restrained eater is a fad dieter who wants to eat her favorite food but will not allow herself to eat it. She is under constant pressure to "be good" and struggles with her willpower to not eat too many calories, break her cleanse, or go over her points. She eliminates certain categories of food from the daily intake—these are known as the forbidden foods. A restrained eater often has a very slow metabolism due to restricting her meals to very low-calorie foods. When this fad dieter finally caves in, she eats ferociously. Women who are restrained eaters have lost the ability to honor their internal hunger and fullness cues. Are you a restrained eater? Don't worry, because you're about to apply the Five Pillars of Positive Nutrition from Chapter 4, eating according to a certain meal structure while giving your body the opportunity to reset the hunger and fullness cycle.

External eating means eating for reasons other than internal hunger cues. You're altering your eating in an effort to reach external goals, such as a certain number of calories, points, or grams of carbohydrates, or even a particular weight on your bathroom scale. Eating for these external reasons rather than in response to internal cues does not honor your biological needs. I know this sounds negative. But taken to extremes, this type of external eating can lead to something known as binge-eating disorder.

However, external eating can also be positive when it's not too low in calories or too restrictive. External eating that teaches adequate consumption and permits all foods can be an amazing tool. This type of external eating can be useful for a short period of time—for example, as we will use it during Phase 1.

Meal Structure Is a Healthy Use of External Eating

How can you eat for external reasons and help yourself? By implementing the Body Clock Diet Phase 1 meal structure for 2 weeks; it tells you what to eat, when to eat, and how much to eat. As mentioned above, you will be eating three meals and two

WHAT IS METABOLIC SYNDROME?

Metabolic syndrome is an umbrella term for a cluster of health conditions such as high blood pressure, high cholesterol, high blood sugar, insulin resistance, and significant abdominal fat that are associated with heart disease, stroke, and diabetes. To lower your risk, the All Foods Fit philosophy will likely help. A study in the *Journal of Nutrition* found that consuming a greater variety of nutrient-packed foods was linked to less belly fat and a decreased risk of high blood pressure. By eating all foods in moderation, you will be more likely to eat a greater diversity of whole foods that deliver the nutrition you need and automatically limit the processed foods linked to metabolic syndrome.

snacks a day. This will never change. The meals and snacks are the roman numerals on an outline. The foods at each meal will change and increase in variety over time. The portions are set in the first few weeks but will eventually be determined by your internal belly-brain cues. This will ensure that you overcome restrained eating because you have enough food and eat frequently enough.

The meal structure will stabilize your blood sugar and your insulin and even help you reclaim your body clock's ability to synchronize hunger and fullness. External eating is recommended only when applied in this way.

Mindful Eating

Eventually—in the next 6 weeks—you will become a mindful eater. You will be aware of mealtimes and snack times. You will connect with your internal rhythms to determine how much food you need to eat. You will be fully present at each meal because you'll use your breath before even starting a meal. You will identify which type of hunger you're feeling and how you want to act. You may choose to eat or use a skill to overcome a craving that is not a true biological need.

To achieve mindful eating, you will start logging your food and feelings in Phase 1. At first you'll log the food you consume and why you consume it, identifying which type of hunger you're experiencing. You'll become aware of how the food you eat affects your fullness, your energy, your mood, and your GI tract. Mindful eating is eating breakfast because it's truly the most important meal of the day, even if you're not hungry. You'll learn that if you skip breakfast, you'll overeat at lunch or get hungry in your morning meeting, eating two doughnuts because they taste good but don't fill you. Eating mindfully is recognizing that you physically need fuel, and all foods provide calories—thus, fuel.

Why Less Is More

Think about what you ate over the past 2 weeks. Did you eat the same breakfast most mornings? The same lunch? What about dinner? In my nutrition practice, most clients tell me they eat the same foods daily because it's part of their habit. They know what's easy and what they think works. Fewer choices are sometimes more. In the spirit of less is more, we give you three options for each meal with three corresponding recipes. This gives you choice but keeps things simple. And we all know simple is best and leads to easy success.

To make things easier, most of our recipes are made for one or two servings—one for breakfast and lunch and two for dinner. (If there are four servings, share with friends or freeze for a meal option in a different phase.) Save the second portion of your dinner meal for later in the week. It will save time, decision making, and effort. Each week, there are at least two servings of fish to boost your intake of

BINGE EATING AS A DISORDER

What is binge eating, and could you possibly have binge-eating disorder (BED)? First of all, a binge is basically eating a large amount of food over a short period of time and feeling out of control, guilty, and perhaps even numb. Unfortunately, this is more common than you might think. According to statistics from the National Association of Anorexia and Associated Disorders, BED occurs in 1 out of every 35 adults in the United States. This means that about 5 million women have BED. I honestly think this number is even higher, and with greater education and awareness, the numbers will jump dramatically. Years ago I volunteered at a *Women's Health* magazine event in New York City, and 37 out of the 40 women I educated on nutrition reported bingeing. Many times what starts out as a fad diet or restrained eating becomes deprivation. By the end of the day, women feel so restricted and starved, they binge to satisfy extreme physical hunger and are unable to control it.

This is why it's so important to train yourself to eat mindfully and remain observant of your dietary habits. If you note out-of-control behaviors around food after limiting your calories, you're receiving a clear warning message that your body needs more food. Going on a binge doesn't necessarily mean you have BED. BED is accompanied by other characteristics of eating disorders such as anorexia and bulimia. But if you suspect you have an eating disorder or BED, seek your doctor's help and reach out for additional information from the Binge Eating Disorder Association (BEDA) and National Eating Disorders Association (NEDA). Resources are identified on page 249.

essential omega-3 fatty acids, decreasing inflammation caused by stress and aiding in better nerve transmission.

The first option you'll find is the Make Me option to make at home. Take the time, follow the recipe, and learn your way around your kitchen using your favorite ingredients.

The second meal option is called Time Crunch. This meal can be easily made ahead of time. For example, follow the recipe for Turkey Chili (page 144), portion it, and freeze the leftovers for the second week of Phase 1. Heat the other portion later in the week for dinner or whenever you are crunched for time.

A third option called Eat In or Out is also included in your meal structure. You can purchase this meal outside of your home or just as easily make it at home. An opportunity to eat outside of the home helps foster the lifestyle component of this plan. Being realistic and thinking long-term is essential when developing new lifetime behaviors.

CHAPTER 6

Reset Button #3: Go to Bed Like Clockwork

SEND STRESS (AND CRAVINGS) PACKING AND SETTLE DOWN TO A LONG, REJUVENATING SLUMBER

You've probably heard this 100 times: Getting 7 to 9 hours of quality sleep regularly is one of the best things you can do for your health and your waistline. Dozens of studies show that people with the most variation in sleep duration put on weight, while those with more consistent sleep patterns actually lose weight. And those who put on the pounds tend to deposit fat around the internal organs, the most dangerous kind of weight gain.

Lack of sleep makes us eat more. In one study at the University of Colorado, people ate more carbohydrates and 6 percent more calories during the day when they didn't get enough sleep the night before. Other studies suggest that women are likely to eat more than 250 extra calories per day when they don't get 7 to 8 hours of shut-eye.

Our circadian rhythm, our internal master clock, drives our sleep patterns in response to light and darkness and regulates the timing of periods of sleepiness and alertness throughout the day. When we disrupt those patterns by staying up late or tossing and turning because we had a late-evening coffee, our bodies let us know about it. Our immune systems weaken, opening us up to colds. Habitual poor sleep ages your arteries and puts you at increased risk of heart disease. It gives you bags under your eyes and makes you look tired . . . and older. Lack of good sleep is a libido buster. It fogs the brain. The list goes on and on.

There are so many downsides to getting poor sleep, but the fix is pretty simple. Getting good-quality sleep comes from establishing a pattern, working with your circadian rhythm, and avoiding deviation. In time the body adjusts and begins to operate optimally, which helps you get leaner. Below are step-by-step instructions for pushing Reset Button #3 to realign your master body clock, plus some terrific tips for getting a better night's sleep. You'll also take a quiz that'll help determine if you're a morning person or an evening person (as if you didn't know already). Take it anyway; it'll either confirm what you know or surprise you.

PRESS HERE FOR GOOD SLEEP

You already know your main body clock demands rest during the dark cycle and activity during the light cycle. So over the next 6 weeks, I want you to adhere to sleeping with the natural *diurnal* cycle based on a single 24-hour rotation of Earth. Here are the steps that will ensure you get restful, rejuvenating, clock-resetting sleep.

1. CUT OFF THE CAFFEINE. The stimulant can stay in your system for 4 or more hours. So avoid coffee, tea, and other caffeinated beverages after 3:00 p.m. Same goes for chocolate, which contains caffeine. If you find yourself still buzzed at bedtime, experiment with cutting off caffeine at noon.

2. TAKE A WALK ON THE BRIGHT SIDE. Your job may stunt your nighttime slumber, especially if you work in a windowless environment. A study at Northwestern University found that people who were employed in offices that lacked sunlight slept 47 fewer minutes a night, on average, than those with office windows. Why? You know the answer; it's the zeitgeber light! Natural light streaming through your optic nerves and hitting the SCN cells synchronizes your circadian clock, enhancing your production of the sleep hormone melatonin at night. But don't quit your job. You can nudge things back to normal by simply taking a half-hour walk out-doors during your lunch break.

3. LIMIT ALCOHOL. Yes, they call it a nightcap, and yes, alcohol can make you drowsy. But booze is also a well-documented sleep destroyer. If you want a good night's sleep, especially during the Body Clock Diet phases, cut out happy hour and go for an early-evening run instead.

4. DESTRESS AND OCCUPY. The period between dinnertime and bedtime is the most dangerous time of day for eating additional calories due to behavioral and emotional hunger. During Phases 1 and 2, self-care tools like journaling, using

BREATHING LESSONS
Master the Dirgha, or Complete Breath,
to Calm the Mind and Enhance Awareness

Pranayama Dirgha, or the Complete Breath, is a three-part breathing technique that's done prior to meditation, but it can be used at any time to eliminate stress and help you focus on the moment. This technique was taught to me by Kripalu-certified yoga teacher and eating disorder expert Susan Schrott, LCSW, CEDS, of New York City. Here is my interpretation for you.

- Close your mouth. Breathe through your nose.
- Take a deep and big breath starting in your belly, allowing your belly, front, sides, and back to expand.
- Work your way up, breathing into your chest cavity, expanding your ribs and back until you reach your throat. This is all one breath that literally moves from the belly up to the throat, oxygenating all your organs, aiding in digestion, and filling you with positive energy.
- Exhale slowly through your nose, first releasing the air in your throat area, your chest cavity, and finally your belly.
- Give yourself a little smile! You did it. Repeat your breath and sit quietly. You can let your mind wander; just be aware of whatever it's focusing on. Notice it and let it go.

your comfort card, painting, practicing music, and so on can soothe stress and distract you from thoughts of food. Exercise is also excellent for quelling non-physical hunger. Just don't exercise vigorously too close to bedtime. Too much activity late at night will heat your body, making it difficult to settle into a sleep rhythm. Also, exercise at night can delay melatonin release so it's harder to wind down. Yoga, stretching, light exercise, and breathing techniques (try the Dirgha breath on page 63) are all good exercises that won't disturb sleep. And I'm an advocate of rigorous exercise too, provided it's done early in the evening. Overall, frequent exercise eases anxiety and limits weight gain, both of which can contribute to sleep trouble, especially in your forties and fifties.

5. DVR JIMMY KIMMEL. Go to bed early enough that you will not need an alarm to wake up. What time is that? Well, you have to experiment a bit. One way to do that is to go to bed 15 minutes earlier than you did last night and see how you feel in the morning. Keep hitting the feathers 15 minutes earlier until you find your sweet spot.

6. DEEP-SIX THE ALARM. Ideally, go to bed early enough that you will not need an alarm clock to wake you but instead will wake naturally according to your body clock. You should try to average 8 hours of sleep per night.

7. GO TO BED AT THE SAME TIME EVERY NIGHT. And wake up at the same time every day. This ensures that sleep becomes habitual, because we do know the body clock works best when it's expecting timed cues from food, light, and stress.

8. KEEP THE ELECTRONICS OFF THE BED. Countless sleep experts agree that you should train yourself to associate your bed with only two things: sleeping and sex. If you watch TV there, check e-mail, or do computer work, suddenly the sleep zone becomes the work and/or entertainment zone and you may have trouble getting to sleep. What's more, the blue light of electronic gadgets can confuse your brain about whether it's night or day.

 Ticktock Tip

Listen to Mozart or the Beatles' "I'm So Tired" to get into the rhythm of slumber. Researchers at Case Western Reserve University say that listening to music in the 60 to 80 beats per minute range, which is a close match to your resting heartbeat, promotes more satisfying and restful sleep.

9. MAKE IT BLACK AND COOL. Your body clock naturally causes a lowering of your core temperature at night to signal oncoming sleep. But if you keep your bedroom too warm, your internal clock may think it's time to rise, and this will disturb your sleep. Optimum room temperature for falling asleep is around 72°F, according to sleep scientists. And be aware of wool blankets and fluffy down comforters. They can bake you like a potato and screw up your sleep.

10. STAY IN BED. Don't let your mind wander out of bed and over to tomorrow or this past afternoon. Think of something fun to distract yourself from the stresses of the day and the to-do list of the day ahead. Phases 1 through 3 identify this time of day as Project Self. This is when you will dedicate time to use tools, exercise, and even begin meditation. See Chapters 7 through 11.

EARLY BIRDS VERSUS NIGHT OWLS

Are you a woman who likes to rise and shine or are you a night owl? Take the morning/evening questionnaire below to help identify your body clock's tendencies. Though not definitive, they may have something to do with your weight struggles. Circle the number below your chosen answer and add those numbers for your score.

1. What time would you get up if you were entirely free to plan your day?

5:00–6:30 a.m.	6:30–7:45 a.m.	7:45–9:45 a.m.	9:45–11:00 a.m.	11:00 a.m.– 12:00 noon	12:00 noon– 5:00 p.m.
5	4	3	2	1	0

2. What time would you go to bed if you were entirely free to plan your evening?

8:00–9:00 p.m.	9:00–10:15 p.m.	10:15 p.m.– 12:30 a.m.	12:30–1:45 a.m.	1:45–3:00 a.m.	3:00–8:00 a.m.
5	4	3	2	1	0

3. If there is a specific time at which you have to get up in the morning, to what extent do you depend on being woken up by an alarm clock?

Not at all dependent	Slightly dependent	Fairly dependent	Very dependent
4	3	2	1

4. How easy do you find it to get up in the morning (when you are not woken up unexpectedly)?

Not at all easy	Not very easy	Fairly easy	Very easy
1	2	3	4

5. How alert do you feel during the first half hour after you wake up in the morning?

Not at all alert	Slightly alert	Fairly alert	Very alert
1	2	3	4

6. How hungry do you feel during the first half hour after you wake up in the morning?

Not at all hungry	Slightly hungry	Fairly hungry	Very hungry
1	2	3	4

7. During the first half hour after you wake up in the morning, how tired do you feel?

Very tired	Fairly tired	Fairly refreshed	Very refreshed
1	2	3	4

8. If you have no commitments the next day, what time do you go to bed compared to your usual bedtime?

Seldom or never later	Less than 1 hour later	1 to 2 hours later	More than 2 hours later
4	3	2	1

9. You have decided to engage in some physical exercise. A friend suggests that you do this for 1 hour twice a week, and the best time for him is between 7:00 and 8:00 a.m. Bearing in mind nothing but your own internal "clock," how do you think you would perform?

Would be in good form	Would be in reasonable form	Would find it difficult	Would find it very difficult
4	3	2	1

10. At what time of day do you feel you become tired as a result of need for sleep?

8:00–9:00 p.m.	9:00–10:15 p.m.	10:15 p.m.–12:45 a.m.	12:45–2:00 a.m.	2:00–3:00 a.m.
5	4	3	2	1

11. You want to be at your peak performance for a test you know is going to be mentally exhausting and will last for 2 hours. Considering only your own internal "clock," which ONE of the four testing times would you choose?

8:00–10:00 a.m.	11:00 a.m.–1:00 p.m.	3:00–5:00 p.m.	7:00–9:00 p.m.
1	2	3	4

12. If you got into bed at 11:00 p.m., how tired would you be?

Not at all tired	A little tired	Fairly tired	Very tired
1	2	3	4

13. For some reason you have gone to bed several hours later than usual, but there is no need to get up at any particular time the next morning. Which ONE of the following are you most likely to do?

Will wake up at usual time but will NOT fall back asleep	Will wake up at usual time and will doze thereafter	Will wake up at usual time but will fall asleep again	Will NOT wake up until later than usual
4	3	2	1

14. One night you have to remain awake between 4:00 and 6:00 a.m to carry out a night watch. You have no commitments the next day. Which ONE of the alternatives will suit you best?

Would NOT go to bed until watch was over	Would take a nap before and sleep after	Would take a good sleep before and nap after	Would sleep only before watch
1	2	3	4

(continued)

15. You have to do 2 hours of hard physical work. You are entirely free to plan your day. Considering only your own internal "clock," which one of the following times would you choose?

8:00–10:00 a.m.	11:00 a.m.–1:00 p.m.	3:00–5:00 p.m.	7:00–9:00 p.m.
4	3	2	1

16. Suppose you can choose your own work hours. Assume that you work a 5-hour day (including breaks) and that your job is interesting and pays by results. Which 5 consecutive hours would you select?

5 hours starting between 4:00 and 8:00 a.m.	5 hours starting between 8:00 and 9:00 a.m.	5 hours starting between 9:00 a.m. and 2:00 p.m.	5 hours starting between 2:00 and 5:00 p.m.	5 hours starting between 5:00 p.m. and 4:00 a.m.
5	4	3	2	1

17. At what time of the day do you think you reach your "feeling best" peak?

5:00–8:00 a.m.	8:00–10:00 a.m.	10:00 a.m.–5:00 p.m.	5:00–10:00 p.m.	10:00 p.m.–5:00 a.m.
5	4	3	2	1

18. One hears about "morning" and "evening" types of people. Which ONE of these types do you consider yourself to be?

Definitely a "morning" type	Rather more a "morning" than an "evening" type	Rather more an "evening" than a "morning" type	Definitely an "evening" type
6	4	2	0

Adapted from J. A. Horne and O. Ostberg (1976), "A Self Assessment Questionnaire to Determine Morningness to Eveningness in Human Circadian Rhythms," *International Journal of Chronobiology* 4: 97–110.

People scoring under 53 are considered "night owls," staying up late at night and sleeping late in the morning, while those scoring above 64 are "early birds" and prefer going to bed early and rising with the sun. If you fall between the two extremes, scoring a 53 to 64, you are neutral. Most people are neutral.

Knowing your bird type can help determine your optimal time to go to sleep and to wake. If you find you are a night owl, recognize that your bedtime may need to be reined in. It doesn't mean you need to go to bed when Grandma does; rather it means your peak rhythms will be slightly later in the day than a morning person's. In Phase 1, the structure uses 7:00 a.m. as a wake-up time. If you're a night owl, you may need to consider your late tendencies and plan for a later wake-up time of 8:00 or 9:00 a.m. yet earlier than your usual wake-up time. Also, recognize that night owl behaviors may make you more susceptible to health issues similar to those of a shift worker. Be sure to recognize whether this is just a function of your lifestyle (i.e., you're a college student, singleton, or shift worker) or it's part of your DNA (for example, from diapers till now, your best time of day has been late evening).

THE BASICS OF BEGINNING THE RESET

To reset your body clock, you must engage all three reset buttons. This is exactly what you'll do over the next 2 weeks. Phase 1 is the foundation for your body clock. As you learned in Chapter 4 and in this chapter, you'll be living and breathing Reset #1, the Five Pillars of Positive Nutrition, identifying your hunger type, and using the tools based on your eating behavior. Then, for Reset #2, you follow a well-defined eating structure to get your body back on track using the three macronutrients—protein, fat, and carbohydrate—and the biological cycles governed by the 24-hour body clock. Your day covers everything from morning through night, including Reset #3, creating a habitual sleep process.

If you have any history of dieting, even during childhood, there is a chance that your biological process of hunger is probing you to gain more and more weight. If you have gained weight from overeating, for emotional and behavioral reasons or just because highly palatable foods override your fullness signals, you're moving to a tune not originally meant for your body or mind. That's why you're reading this book—you want to reset your body clock! Welcome to Phase 1 of the *Women's Health* Body Clock Diet. Give yourself a hug, turn to the next chapter, and begin living again.

Part III

BODY CLOCK REPAIR

and

Maintenance

CHAPTER
7

Phase 1: Reset Your Clock

TAKE 2 WEEKS TO RESYNCHRONIZE YOUR BODY CLOCK AND START LOSING WEIGHT

L et's start getting back into rhythm. In Phase 1 of the Body Clock Diet, you'll punch three key reset buttons to resynchronize your circadian rhythm, your master body clock. This critical phase lasts 2 weeks. Resetting your clock is the first step toward boosting your metabolism and actually losing weight. It will provide fast, positive feedback and help you begin structuring your meals into a rhythm of regular fueling to avoid the sabotaging trap of ravenous hunger.

In this chapter, you'll find four guiding principles and an hour-by-hour recommended daily schedule that will help recalibrate your body clock. In addition, you'll learn how to use a key tool I suggest for my clients called a mindful meal log. You'll find a sample on page 82 and blank meal log pages to fill out at the end of this chapter. You'll use this log as you progress into Phases 2 and 3 as well. Think of it as your 6-week travel diary as you establish a pattern of healthy living for life!

FIND YOUR SHADOW

Famed psychologist Carl G. Jung wrote, "To confront a person with his shadow is to show him his own light." The shadow is that part of us that's often beyond the threshold of our awareness. The mindful meal log reveals your shadow. It's a tool to help you become your own body detective, a simple way for you to become mindful of the fact that you often eat for reasons other than pure, empty-belly hunger.

The act of recording the foods you eat and writing down your feelings makes them tangible. Logs like this help us to note our patterns, whether they're helpful or detrimental. Don't worry. This is not something you'll have to do for the rest of your life. But it's a terrific exercise to use during the 6-week Body Clock Diet program.

Your log will help you identify what meals are eaten for emotional, behavioral, or physical reasons while also presenting an unbiased record of which foods fill you, fatigue you, or trigger overeating. It'll be an eye-opener, I guarantee!

Skip a meal? This log will show you in black and white what happens and how you'll feel as a result. It will be evident if poor sleep or too little sleep triggers a greater appetite. This information is for you only. Be completely honest as you journal your food and eating/hunger types over the next 2 weeks.

GUIDELINES FOR PHASE 1

YOUR WATER: Start each morning off with a mug of warm water. (Add a squeeze of lemon if you like.) The heat will stimulate the gastrointestinal tract to aid in digestion and trigger peristalsis for bowel movements to keep you regular.

YOUR WINE: Avoid alcoholic beverages completely in Phase 1. Alcohol disrupts circadian rhythm and digestion, and it may make you hungrier. While wine can be heart protective, all alcoholic beverages are likely to add belly fat. Cutting out cocktails for 2 weeks is one of the smartest things you can do to lose weight.

YOUR COFFEE: Coffee in moderation is okay. This means one or two cups daily before 2:00 p.m. to prevent sleep interference and spikes of the stress hormone.

YOUR SUGAR: Skip the artificial sweeteners. Eat the real deal. Artificial sugar can upset the stomach and actually desynchronize your circadian rhythm by confusing your body; the sweet taste makes your brain think you're bringing in calories when you're not. Skip the diet drinks and sugar-free foods, too. Eat real.

DAYS 1 TO 14
Your Hour-by-Hour Stop (Gaining Weight) Watch

Follow this time schedule to reset your body to a natural rhythm that optimizes your biological processes. To recap: The Body Clock Diet is not a fad diet that promises rapid weight loss. Remember that as appealing as crazy-fast results may seem, they're actually detrimental to long-term success. If you drop more than 10 percent of your current body weight in the first 2 weeks, you have the potential to decrease your metabolism. Think: Slow and steady wins the race.

6:00 to 7:00 a.m.—Rise and Shine with the Sun

Pop out of bed right away. Don't hit the snooze button, because drifting into a new sleep cycle and waking up again can disrupt your normal Z's pattern, and you'll drag your butt the rest of the day. If it's wintertime and still pitch dark outside at 6:00, you might want to sleep in until sunlight starts peeking through your shades. Sunlight governs our circadian rhythm. The idea here is to rise with light to resync your body clock and also to go to bed and wake up at roughly the same time every day. This creates sleep habituation, a crucial part of the body clock reset. For the next 2 weeks I want you to go to bed and wake at the same time, allowing for a solid 8 hours of sleep. So if you're going to rise with the sun at 6:00, that means

 Ticktock Tip

Lighten Up!

To speed up your body clock reset, try to get outdoors soon after you wake up. Research shows that spending 30 to 45 minutes outside in natural light can nudge a whacked-out circadian rhythm in the right direction. Just leave your sunglasses inside. Your eyes and brain need to absorb that natural light to work the magic. You should find that after a few days of morning exposure to UV light, you'll feel sleepier at night and brighter the following mornings. If you can't get outside for some reason (or live in Alaska), try sitting in front of a sunlamp.

hitting the feathers by 10:00 p.m. Now don't stress if rising at 6:00 a.m. is not manageable for you. Just make sure you achieve 7 to 9 hours of quality sleep and try to wake with the sun as best you can. The goal is to wake during the light and sleep during the dark cycle of the 24-hour period.

7:00 a.m.—Get Your Groove On

Around 7:00 a.m. your cortisol is peaking, so take advantage of this boost in alertness by getting moving. Shower, dress, get ready for your day, and if you have children, get them up and ready for school. You don't need caffeine or carbs yet. Your already high cortisol gives you the needed edge, while caffeine and carbs would cause a double-whammy surge in both insulin and blood sugar. In other words, they set you up for diabetes!

8:00 a.m.—Time to Eat

Hold on. Before grabbing your fork, grab your mindful meal log (see sample on page 82) so you can write in it before and after your meal. Be sure to record how many hours you slept and how you feel. Are you thinking about food? Are you hungry? Can you tell if it's emotional, behavioral, or physical hunger?

You should eat breakfast about an hour after waking. (So if you rose at 6:00 instead of 7:00, you'll want to eat a little earlier than 8:00 a.m.) An hour after rising will be ideal, because your cortisol levels will be decreasing. This will allow the body to respond to your breakfast rather than cortisol and breakfast (the double-whammy effect). Your insulin will increase to lower your blood sugar, and leptin will be released to let your belly-brain know it's fed.

Breakfast Choices

Choose from the following three meal selections. You may continue to use these recipes as part of your lifestyle. Rotate through the three meal choices for the next 2 weeks.

- **MAKE ME:** Avocado Toast (page 132)

- **TIME CRUNCH:** Peanut Butter Overnight Oats (page 131)

- **EAT IN OR OUT:** Greek yogurt with KIND Healthy Grains Maple Quinoa Clusters with Chia Seeds (1 cup). (This granola has inulin in it. Belly bacteria love

The Argument for Never Skipping Breakfast

Many women eat tiny breakfasts or no breakfast at all because they feel that's being "a good dieter." Well, research says otherwise. A high-protein, high-carbohydrate, and high-calorie breakfast has been shown to result in lower blood sugar, decreased insulin resistance, and decreased production of the hormone ghrelin that stimulates appetite later in the afternoon. This breakfast may even prevent weight gain!

to feed on it. When attempting to create a healthier microbiome, the inulin, which is basically a soluble fiber, acts as a prebiotic, which will work well with the probiotics from the Greek yogurt.) Be sure to add granola gradually, because inulin (a polysaccharide) can cause gas and bloating.

9:00 a.m.—Coffee Safe!

You've had a protein-packed breakfast meal and made it to the office. Yes, you can have coffee now. We're talking lifestyle, ladies! I would never ask you to do something I don't do. And I do drink coffee. Drink your coffee now while the hormone cortisol is lower. It can help you get the extra edge to deal with the day ahead. One to two cups of coffee daily is just fine. But remember to avoid artificial sugars. Use real sugar and cream or half and half, if you like. Or wean yourself off the sweetener and the dairy and enjoy the full, natural flavor of a good roasted coffee taken black.

10:00 a.m.—Savory Selections

Grab that pen again and log before and after your midmorning snack. For the first 2 weeks, I suggest a midmorning snack and an afternoon snack. Eating every 2 hours in Phase 1 is extremely helpful when overcoming overeating and restrictive or "restrained eating," a nutritionists' term for limiting calories to lose weight. Choose one of the three savory snacks below to help decrease the desire to eat for hedonic reasons.

- 1 orange and 16 nuts

- 1 apple and ¼ cup hummus

- 3 mini pitas and 16 pitted olives

12:00 noon—Lunchtime

Again, log before and after this meal. If you ate a large breakfast high in protein as recommended and had a smart snack midmorning, you won't be ravenous at lunchtime. In fact, you're probably still busy with work at this time. That's okay. Lunch can be anytime between noon and 2:30 but never after. If you're busy and expect a late lunch, just switch your afternoon snack with your lunch. This means you would eat your afternoon snack sometime shortly after noon and lunch by 2:30 p.m. at the latest. Research indicates that eating lunch before 3:00 p.m. equals greater weight loss. This may be related to a specific body clock gene.

Visit page 135 for some suggestions for Phase 1 lunches. I know how busy your days can get, so I've built in some Time Crunch options you can prepare ahead of time and easily pack if you're short on time and some Eat Out options you can purchase at a local deli, diner, or even fast-food restaurant. See the following examples. Try all the three lunch options throughout the week, as this will help make these foods part of your habitual nourishment. Eating a variety of foods ensures you get all the vitamins and minerals you need and keeps your clock ticking.

- **MAKE ME:** Sunny Bowl: Eggs over Mashed Butternut Squash and Kale (page 138). Easy cooking is part of your new lifestyle! Make this recipe ahead and just heat before you eat.

- **TIME CRUNCH:** Peanut Butter 'n' Berry Sandwich with Greek Yogurt (page 135). This is an easy staple and a childhood favorite. Enjoy!

- **EAT IN OR OUT:** Spinach salad. This salad option is easy to make or purchase. Add your choice of protein, either chicken, turkey, or fish.

3:30 p.m.—Tame Temptation Time

At about this time in the afternoon, cortisol, insulin, and blood sugar decrease, leaving you feeling lethargic and often craving sugar. Choose one of the three savory snacks below. (Remember to log before and after the snack.)

- 2 tablespoons dark chocolate chips and one 0.6-ounce Barney's Almond Butter Squeeze (90 calories)

- Beets and goat cheese (½ cup beets, canned, drained, with 1 ounce goat cheese)

- Skinny Pop popcorn (individual bag) and 2 Laughing Cow Mini Babybel cheeses

Enjoy your snack and then get moving to increase your alertness. This is a very precarious time. Don't fall prey to behavioral eating or reach for sugar and coffee to perk you up. Rather, step outside to increase cortisol naturally. Walk for 5 minutes, or if you can't bear to leave the office or house, try a few yoga exercises in your chair to increase your energy by pumping oxygen throughout your body. Use the Tame Temptation Tools below.

6:30 p.m.—Dinnertime!

What are you going to do? That's right: Log before and after the meal. For optimum weight maintenance and to make your body clock hum more efficiently, try to consume the majority of your calories early in the day. That's why I advocate a sizable breakfast including protein, fat, and carbs. If you've had a hearty breakfast and have been eating something every 3 to 4 hours over the course of the day, you'll reach dinnertime with a belly that's ready to eat but not so hungry you'll eat half a baguette before your meal has finished cooking!

Tame Temptation Tools

1. Eat moderate carbs with protein and fat at lunch to prevent a blood sugar roller coaster that ends in an even more fatiguing slump between 3:00 and 4:00 p.m.

2. Strike a yoga pose such as Warrior 1, 2, or 3.

3. Ride it out with a power nap (10 minutes max).

4. Listen to your favorite tunes.

5. Walk it off (10 minutes to combat sleepiness).

6. Feel free to caffeinate (as long as it doesn't affect your sleep cycle).

THE BENEFITS OF MIXING MACRONUTRIENTS

The mixed meal is for optimal blood sugar. When you eat a carbohydrate, the body releases insulin to act as the transfer agent. Insulin transfers carbohydrates, aka sugar/starch, to your cells by connecting to the insulin receptor site. The cell door opens to allow the carb/sugar into the cell to create energy. Complicated, right? Well, all you need to know is that the more carbohydrates you eat, the more insulin is released. Eat too many carbs, and your body can eventually become insulin resistant. Another term for this is *prediabetes*, the precursor to full-blown type 2 diabetes.

To prevent this from happening, be sure your meals and snacks contain a mix of the macronutrients protein, fat, and carbohydrate. If you eat protein and fat with the sugar (carbs), it will take your body longer to break down and absorb the complex combination of all three macronutrients. In effect, the combo meal lowers the glycemic load of the food. The sugar gets released slowly into your blood—no blood sugar spikes!—so the body no longer needs a flood of insulin to deal with all that sugar. Here are two great mixed-meal examples: deli turkey (protein) on whole grain bread (carbs) with sliced avocado (fat); and stir-fried vegetables (carbs) with tofu (protein) and peanuts (fat and protein).

Take a look at the suggested Phase 1 dinner recipes starting on page 140. There are enough so you won't get bored with the meals. I included one of my faves, a ground turkey and bean chili. This is a terrific Phase 1 meal because it's high in lean protein (from the turkey and beans), belly-filling fiber (again, the beans), and vitamin-rich vegetables. You'll find that one serving is very satisfying. You probably won't be hungry for an evening snack after this dinner, which will make it even easier for you to get into wind-down mode for the night. This dish makes four servings, so you can polish off two with your dinner partner and have two leftover portions to freeze for next week or for take-to-work lunches. Learn to use leftovers wisely. They're efficient, they'll save you money, and they'll reduce the number of times you opt for takeout. Here are a few of the dinner options you'll find in Chapter 12.

- **MAKE ME:** Spaghetti Squash and Meatballs (page 140)

- **MAKE ME:** Chipotle Pork Tenderloin with Baby Kale Salad (page 142)

- **TIME CRUNCH:** Turkey Chili (page 144)

- **EAT IN OR OUT:** Order 5 ounces protein, 1 cup grain, and 2 cups veggies

8:00 p.m.—Project Self

This is a time I want you to carve out for just you. If you have kids, get them into bed before tackling this project. If it's only you at home, then make sure you've finished the dishes and are ready for you time. Here's the thinking behind Project Self: The time between 8:00 and 10:00 p.m. is a well-documented temptation time zone when a lot of people reach for the pint of ice cream or bag of chips out of boredom or in response to carbohydrate cravings before bed. Project Self is designed to outsmart those temptations by occupying your hands and attention with something constructive and calorie-free. Remember your comfort card and Boot Behavioral Eating tips? Grab them and lose yourself in your hobby or pastime. This is an important part of your body clock reset. Basically you'll be creating a new after-dinner habit to replace the mindless snacking that disrupts your circadian rhythm.

10:00 or 11:00 p.m.—Your Mini Meditation

Normally, the stress hormone naturally decreases at this time of night to make you sleepy, but if your body clock is out of kilter, cortisol may still be coursing through your body, keeping you on high alert and making it difficult to wind down and get that full 8 hours of restful sleep your body needs.

One proven technique for reducing cortisol is meditation. You'll learn a simple meditation exercise in Chapter 10, but if you aren't used to meditating or find the idea a little intimidating, before bed during Phase 1, try a simple 1-minute meditation prompted by an easy breathing technique. This three-part yoga breath taught to me by Susan Schrott, a Kripalu-certified yoga teacher, is known as Dirgha breath. I've adapted it slightly for the beginner. See "Breathing Lessons" on page 63.

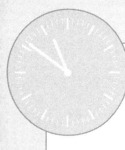

PHASE 1 SAMPLE MINDFUL MEAL LOG

By understanding how and why you eat, you'll become a more mindful eater. And you will see in black and white why it's so much easier to lose weight by eating high-quality food at regular intervals versus starving yourself and counting calories. This is a sample log that's been filled out by one of my clients. Use this as a guide to filling out your own daily meal record in the blank log pages that follow. Think of this as your diary for rebooting your natural biorhythms.

MORNING CHECK-IN:

Wake-Up Time	Hours Slept	Quality of Sleep	Feelings, Thoughts, Behaviors
7 a.m.	6.5	Poor, tossed and turned all night.	Tired; need to get to work on time. Wish there was more time in day.

Time	Type of Hunger	Feelings, Thoughts, Behaviors Before	Food Eaten	Feelings, Thoughts, Behaviors After
BREAKFAST				
8 a.m.	Emotional (Behavioral) (Physical)	I ate because I know I need to; also because I'm starving and I have a morning meeting and don't want my stomach to grumble.	One packet oatmeal with coffee	I still feel hungry. Wish I had more time to make breakfast.
MIDMORNING SNACK				
10:30 a.m.	Emotional Behavioral (Physical)	Finally got more food post meeting	Coffee and Greek yogurt	Finally feel full

Time	Type of Hunger	Feelings, Thoughts, Behaviors Before	Food Eaten	Feelings, Thoughts, Behaviors After
LUNCH				
1:15 p.m.	(Emotional) Behavioral (Physical)	Hungry and anxious. Will be sure to get enough food so this doesn't turn into a binge	Salad from deli with greens, turkey, beans, quinoa, and balsamic dressing	I am overfull but know it is really temporary belly distention from the fiber in the greens, beans and quinoa.
TEMPTATION TIME				
4 p.m.	(Emotional) Behavioral Physical	Feeling tired and need pick-me-up	Cereal bar	I need a protein with this. It doesn't hurt my belly but it is not enough to hold me until dinner.
DINNER				
7 p.m.	Emotional Behavioral (Physical)	Starving and feel like I will overeat	Chili with a side salad. Iced tea, sweetened with lemon and sugar.	That meal was super filling and I didn't overeat. Feel confident that I can turn my life around.

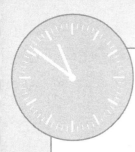

PHASE 1
MINDFUL MEAL LOG

MORNING CHECK-IN:

Wake-Up Time	Hours Slept	Quality of Sleep	Feelings, Thoughts, Behaviors

Time	Type of Hunger	Feelings, Thoughts, Behaviors Before	Food Eaten	Feelings, Thoughts, Behaviors After
BREAKFAST				
	Emotional Behavioral Physical			
MIDMORNING SNACK				
	Emotional Behavioral Physical			

* Make photocopies of this log.

Time	Type of Hunger	Feelings, Thoughts, Behaviors Before	Food Eaten	Feelings, Thoughts, Behaviors After
LUNCH				
	Emotional Behavioral Physical			
TEMPTATION TIME				
	Emotional Behavioral Physical			
DINNER				
	Emotional Behavioral Physical			

CHAPTER
8

Skill Builder:
How to Eat
an Oreo

MASTER MINDFULNESS AND THE WORLD
IS YOUR NO-WORRIES BUFFET

By now you're well on your way to resetting your body clock, or maybe it's on schedule already. Congratulations! I hope you found the tools like the Five Pillars of Positive Nutrition, the meal structure, the breathing techniques, and the comfort card helpful. Tools and skills are like a long-term battery for your master clock. You can use them all your life to keep your body in rhythm.

Now it's time to learn a new skill that will support the All Foods Fit philosophy. It's called mindfulness or mindful eating, and it will supply you with the strength and willpower to enjoy even the most dangerously decadent foods—those that trigger hedonic eating—without going overboard. In fact, mastering mindful eating can help you eat *less* of *any* food overall and support long-term weight loss, according to a study in the journal *Appetite*.

I ATE A SLEEVE OF GIRL SCOUT COOKIES!

Have you ever uttered those words? Here's how it typically happens: You're trying to be "good," so you swear off high-calorie foods, high-fat foods, carbs, and processed foods. You're doing pretty well operating in restraint mode and feeling good about yourself . . . until you decide to have one Thin Mint Girl Scout cookie, or an Oreo, or [plug in your favorite cookie flavor]. Magically, one freakin' cookie turns into five, and before you know it you're in a robotic race to devour them. You can't stop. One row is gone, and the frenzy continues. You have eaten 12 cookies and do not feel full. I've been there. My clients have been there. You're not alone. This can happen with cupcakes, potato chips, pints of ice cream, whatever particular food rules over you.

If you want to eat an Oreo or any delicious, yummy, highly palatable food that is also likely highly processed or just highly scrumptious with sweetness and/or saltiness, there's a way to do it. But first you need to recognize that you're the underdog here. Snack food manufacturers have made a conscious decision to make their products tempting, tantalizing, and tasty to the tongue and brain. The combinations of salt, fat, mouthwatering flavorings, and textures tickle the reward sensors of your brain, the same areas that are triggered by addictive substances like alcohol, marijuana, and other drugs. The food manufacturers design their snacks to tempt you and never let your body feel full, so you can buy and eat more and more. It makes good business, but not great health. And when your body clock is off-kilter, it's even harder to eat these foods without getting into trouble.

But there's a trick to foiling food makers' evil plans to make you overeat. Actually, there are two tricks. One is easier; the other is a little harder but much more versatile, because it can be used in any situation. Let's start with the nearly foolproof way to enjoy a sensible, satisfying taste of what seems to be a highly addictive food.

Ever notice that a bag of sea salt and vinegar potato chips contains more calories than a piece of grilled chicken breast, yet the chicken breast makes you feel much fuller? After eating the chicken, you don't really feel hungry for another chicken breast, but after you reach the bottom of a bag of chips you can easily scarf another.

The trick to stopping at a small portion of a highly processed food is to make sure you eat a satiating food with it. For example, it's best to eat risotto as a side to steak and green beans. The protein in the steak and the fiber and water content in the green beans fill you up and flip your "I'm stuffed" button so you don't overdo the luscious risotto. You're using food to help your body recognize fullness. Easy! So dole out three small cookies as a dessert and eat them immediately before, with, or even immediately after finishing your hummus sandwich, or you'll run to the pantry to grab the box. So there you have it: Tool #1 for portion management of highly tasty foods is always eating them with a satiating mixed meal.

When Down Is Up

After 6 weeks of mindfulness training, participants in a study reported the following noteworthy changes, according to the journal *Complementary Therapies in Medicine*:

- **26** percent decrease in depression
- **35** percent decrease in anxiety
- **39** percent decrease in hunger
- **43** percent decrease in binge-eating incidents

Tool #2 is learning to become a mindful eater so you can enjoy a sensible portion of a highly palatable or formerly triggering food without the help of a full meal.

How to Eat an Oreo:
Your Mindful Eating Exercise

1. Relax and Breathe

Start with a trip to your pantry or deli to select a favorite soon-to-be-former "indulgence food"—a cookie, a cracker, a chip. But only one! If you're choosing to eat an Oreo or some food around which it seems you cannot control yourself, be sure you eat it with a meal and not as a stand-alone snack.

Next, set the table. Place a plate on the table and the food item on the plate. Sit at the table with your feet flat on the floor. Place the napkin on your lap and rest your forearms and hands on the table.

Take a deep breath. This breath should be so deep that when you inhale, your shoulders rise, like they're about to reach your earlobes. On the exhale, you should feel your shoulders fall back slowly.

2. Initiate a Body Scan

Notice your feet. How do they feel? Push your soles into the ground. Imagine you're a reed in a field. Your feet are your roots, and you're firmly connected to the earth, yet your upper body is flexible and can react spontaneously. This mental image, now translating to your posture, is how I want you to feel about life—you're rooted but flexible with what's happening around you. Now, notice the energy you feel as you push your soles into the ground while pulling your ankles in an upward direction. Feel that resistance? This is the energy that runs through your body. Observe it in your calves by squeezing and releasing your calf muscles. Imagine the energy running through your calves, through your knees, and into your thighs to create the tension and let it go. Now let your knees relax and try to contract and release your thighs. Just notice these parts without judgment.

Follow the energy to your abdomen. Contract your abs and release. Again, just notice and be aware. Getting in touch with how you feel and connecting to your body's muscle functions will help in the next few minutes. Bring your attention to your spine. Notice each vertebra. Imagine you are pushing each one gently into the chair or wall behind you. Follow your vertebrae and your breath up your spine to your shoulders.

Mindful Tip #1
Eliminate Distractions

We live in a world where the ability to multitask is considered résumé-worthy. But eating while working, answering e-mails, or doing other tasks can make you consume more than you need. A study in the *American Journal of Clinical Nutrition* found that people who played solitaire during lunch felt less full than undistracted eaters and ate significantly more when offered cookies just half an hour later. So make your meals about focusing on your food: Banish the TV, iPad, smartphone, or book from the table, period.

Gently push your shoulders into the wall or chair back. Notice how that feels, how you feel. And breathe.

Now imagine you're under the most amazing waterfall. The water is washing the weight off your shoulders, off your body. The water trickles down your upper arms and lower arms and falls off your fingertips. Just notice how all of this feels. Make a fist by tightening and releasing your hands, taking any negative thoughts, feelings, or memories and letting them go each time you release. In your mental image, visually let the negative thoughts fall into the stream and watch them blend into the waters. They are gone, and you can breathe again. Bring your attention to your breath.

Breathe in through your nose for 4 seconds and hold the oxygen for 4 seconds while it swirls through your body, then exhale through your mouth for 4 seconds. Repeat this breath cycle a few more times and then focus your awareness on your head—on your cheeks, ears, and scalp. Just notice your presence. It may be helpful to bring awareness to this part of your body by clenching and releasing your jaw. All the while, observe your presence and, of course, your breath. Notice your lips, eyelids, and the air coming through your nose. Breathe in a long and deep breath, set an intention to be mindful and to honor your body, and release the breath and relax.

Mindful Tip #2
Put Food on Display

When you eat straight out of the bag, what's likely to happen? (1) You don't stop until the container is empty and (2) you have no idea how much you actually inhaled. "People can consume a lot more calories if they're not focused on the food," says Lesley Lutes, PhD, an associate professor of psychology at East Carolina University. "Seeing the food—and the portion size—may actually help you feel more full." So regardless of how much or how little you're eating, use a plate or a bowl. Another trick: Leave a bit of food on your plate. After a while, you will have conditioned your body and mind to stop interpreting an empty plate as a full belly.

3. Engage Your Senses

You're almost ready to take your first bite. But now that you're completely relaxed and in tune with your body, take time to call on your senses. You were given five of them. Really make use of them.

SIGHT: Look at the food you have chosen as it sits on the plate. Don't touch it; just observe. What memory does the food bring up for you? Does it remind you of your childhood? Perhaps it holds some meaning. Does it make you feel excited when you see it? Explore these thoughts.

SOUND: Listen. Can you hear your food? Is it quiet? Is it sizzling? Did you choose a deep-fried Oreo? Does it remind you of a sound?

TOUCH: Pick up your food. What does it feel like? Does it crumble in your hands? Melt? Squish? Is it sticky, smooth, rough, or all of the above? Notice if your body is reacting to these three senses. Be aware of your heart rate.

SMELL: Bring the food to your mouth or your nose to the food. What does it smell like? What does this do to your heart rate? What memories are evoked? Notice your salivation.

TASTE: Finally, take a small bite. Notice your heart rate, your breathing, and your salivation. Is your body tense or relaxed? Does the food taste like you thought it would? Move it around slowly in your mouth with your tongue and notice if it has a different taste in different parts of your mouth—pay close attention. Are you chewing on one side of your mouth? Are you not completely chewing your food?

Swallow, take a breath, and notice your body. Are there food remnants in your mouth? Can you taste the flavor of the food? Take another breath and repeat the five-senses exercise for your next bite. Do this a few times.

Mindful Tip #3
Start Slow

When you're learning to be mindful, it's helpful to first quit the feeding frenzy. One easy way to keep a reasonable pace: Put your utensils down and your hands in your lap between bites. Don't worry—tuning in to your eating experience should eventually become second nature, so you won't be stuck dining at this grandma pace forever.

Ticktock Tip

Be a Food Critic

Take note of the nuance of every flavor and how satisfying each item is. For example, when you bite into a grape, all those juices come out. This is a sensation you'd totally miss if you just stuffed a handful of grapes into your mouth at once. Notice the texture and smell of your snack and the thoughts that come up as you eat.

Now, choose to finish your food, save it for later, or throw it away.

Upon completing this for the first time, you will have successfully had your first mindful food experience! Phase 2 will walk you through this experience again and help you gain competence in eating all foods.

The Art of Breathing Before Meals

The mindful eating exercise above is similar to the one I learned in the late '90s when I went to Ellyn Satter's workshop, "Treating the Dieting Casualty." Ellyn taught our class to "center" and taste our food. She had us take a deep breath before we ate our M&M'S and Wheat Thins. I will never forget that day, as it changed my life. I had an epiphany. I hated M&M'S. I learned that they taste like chemicals if I eat them slowly. I also realized that this method of centering and tasting applies to all foods and all meals. Ellyn had us center before and after the meal. I remember that she explained it as a way to separate from the chaos of the day and be psychologically present to taste and be satisfied with our food.

Since then, I've incorporated the four-square breathing technique that I learned from my beloved Jen G. in my yoga practice here in New York.

I realized this was the perfect tool for many of my clients who hate meditation, fear their own feelings, or are just too anxious to notice their thoughts. They love four-square breathing because the focus is on counting, not thoughts or feelings. Try it.

Breathe in through your nose for 4 seconds, hold the oxygen for 4 seconds while it swirls through your body, and then exhale through your mouth for 4 seconds. Repeat.

CORTISOL CRUSHERS AND OTHER TOOLS

Becoming more mindful not only helps with eating healthier, it's an effective skill for stress control. That's why I recommend mindful activities like yoga and Pilates to my clients. They promote the very opposite of the body's natural "fight, flight, or freeze" stress response. One of my colleagues, Susan Schrott, a certified eating disorder specialist and Kripalu-trained yoga instructor, says yoga practice is about the ability to be in your body, to bring oxygen to the brain, and to stimulate the parasympathetic nervous system, the calming part of the autonomic nervous system. Susan specializes in acceptance commitment therapy, a psychological intervention based on being present and accepting what life brings us. I want you to learn to be in your body and apply it to every movement you do—when you hop on your bike, walk to the river, climb onto the elliptical, or just lie on your couch. I always try to explain to my clients that they need to view and love themselves from the inside out versus outside in. These statements may help you better understand the concept.

You're likely working outside in and therefore against yourself if . . .

- You run to clock miles rather than exude your energy.

- You try to change your body through restriction and deprivation.

- You cannot feel hunger and fullness.

- You have trouble sitting still and feeling.

- You don't do yoga or Pilates because you feel it isn't enough of a cardio workout.

How to begin working inside out and with yourself . . .

- Run to release the energy that comes through your feet and body.

- Look at food as a way to feed and nurture your body so that you feel peaceful to be with yourself.

- Get back to basics with the meal structure to allow your body time to expect food, digest food, and rest.

- Identify what makes you anxious and use a tool to defuse it.

- Use yoga or Pilates to experience a flow of energy coming from within you.

Among the favorite tools I learned from Susan is a stress-defusing technique that I call the Cortisol Crushers. Next time you feel stressed out, inadequate, unsure, or just blue, try these five calming practices.

The Five Cortisol Crushers

1. **Identify and list your most heartfelt values.** For example:

   a. To live an honest life

   b. To be a compassionate partner

   c. To be of service in this universe

   d.

   e.

2. **Recognize that thoughts are simply information.** Remove the judgment. There are no good or bad thoughts. If you have a thought, think about whether it will help you to embrace your values. If not, just notice the thought and change your attention toward what will help you achieve your values.

3. **Imagine you have large luggage pieces.** Fill them with your negative thoughts, feelings, and memories. Zip them up and imagine you're carrying them at the airport. Put the bags filled with distress on the luggage conveyor belt and visualize the bags being taken away, to be packed on a plane and sent far away. You have just gotten rid of your emotional baggage. Do you feel lighter? Now you're left with values.

4. **Imagine you have a TV remote control in your hand and hit the pause button.** You did it. You can pause real life and escape stress by just taking a deep breath. Notice how you feel and hit Play when you're ready.

5. **Send a love letter to yourself.** Mail your mind-body-spirit a love letter thanking it for the thoughts. Susan told me, "Words are words, not what we attach to them. Thank your mind even if the thought was negative." This helps you to move away from the judgment.

READING YOUR HUNGER/FULLNESS FUEL GAUGE

Hunger is a very subjective feeling. Everyone's hunger is slightly different, which is why it can be so difficult to learn how to gauge actual hunger, especially when you've tried every diet known to woman and your cues are off. The meal structure in Phase 1 of this program is designed so that you don't need to rely on hunger/fullness cues—the meals are already portion-controlled and contain the right mix of macronutrients. After the first 2 weeks of the Body Clock Diet program, you're ability to recognize hunger/fullness cues will start to return. To make it easier to define your cues, I recommend trying the following exercise and using the hunger/fullness scale.

Listen to your body. What are the sensations that help you define hunger and the feelings of satiety.

_____

_____

_____

List what you think your hunger cues are.

1. _____

2. _____

3. _____

4. _____

List what you think your fullness cues are.

1. _____

2. _____

3. _____

4. _____

Now, considering those clues you listed, rate your hunger/fullness on a scale of 0 to 10, like the one below. Imagine your stomach is the gas tank of a car, where 0 is "E" for empty, 10 is "F" for full, and "5" is neutral—neither full nor empty. Ideally, you'll want to stay in the range between "3" and "7" on this scale, never at either extreme.

0_____Hungry_____5_____Full_____10

At the start of the Body Clock Diet program, your stomach may be stretched from overeating, so don't bother with the cues exercise and hunger/fullness scale until about 2 weeks into Phase 1, about day 15.

Using the hunger/fullness scale will help you to become adept at recognizing when it is time to refuel and it also will help you to understand how long certain foods in certain amounts will keep you satiated. Eating something every 2 to 3 hours as prescribed in Phase 1 will take the guesswork out of that challenge until you master your cues.

The Hunger Tree

A flowchart for dealing with different hunger types

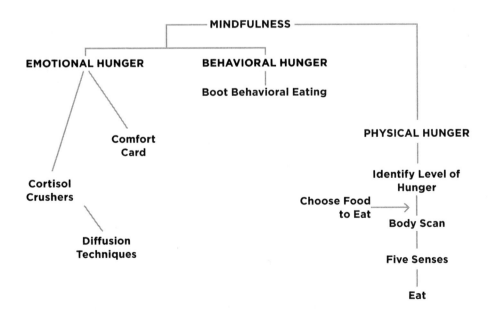

CHAPTER
9

Phase 2: Respect Your Clock

DAYS 15 TO 30: TIME TO FINE-TUNE YOUR CLOCK WITH SELF-CARE

You're 2 weeks into the Body Clock Diet program and the toughest part is just about over. You've learned to use three different types of reset buttons to swing your body clock into proper rhythm. Next, you will refine those practices and turn your focus further inward toward wholeness and healing with self-care. But before we jump into Phase 2 plans, let's review what you've been doing every day.

1. Eating enough calories to keep your metabolism revving high, what we dietitians call "maintaining optimal thermogenesis."

2. Identifying the type of hunger you're experiencing and, if you suspect either emotional or behavioral hunger, using your comfort card, Tame Temptation Tools, and Boot Behavioral Eating to break habitual eating.

3. Reciting the Five Pillars of Positive Nutrition each day.

4. Controlling stress and keeping cortisol low by using the Dirgha breath.

5. Synchronizing circadian rhythm using the Body Clock Diet meal structure and healthy sleep habits.

6. Practicing self-care (through Project Self) and mindfulness techniques.

Now you've reached the point where it's time to "sharpen the saw."

"If you don't sharpen the saw, the saw can't cut." Sometime after college, I believe I read this quote in a book on Buddhism; I reread it years later in Stephen Covey's *The 7 Habits of Highly Effective People.* Covey's seventh habit is "sharpen the saw." Covey relates the story of a man who happens upon a frustrated lumberjack who has been sawing a tree for hours. "Why don't you stop and sharpen the saw?" the man asks. The woodcutter responds, "I don't have time to stop."

The story illustrates a common behavior: Instead of taking time out to develop ourselves and learn to be more efficient and effective, we keep hacking away at life with a dull blade. Sharpening our saw is about the ongoing process of change and self-improvement, and it requires self-respect and self-care.

This is what you'll learn to do in Phase 2: Respect Your Clock, which will lead you from day 15 through day 30. You have learned to identify emotional, behavioral, and physical hunger. You will continue to build upon this new awareness and explore your inner sensations for the cues of hunger and fullness. In the last chapter, you learned how to eat an Oreo using mindfulness and the five senses. Using those tools, your Phase 2 meal structure now includes snack cookies. You see, *all foods really do fit!* Be sure to eat these cookies with lunch. The protein in your sandwich delivers superior satiating powers that will tame your hunger so you can manage a bit of sweetness as a meal ender. Remember to sit quietly, do a body scan, and then proceed to eat mindfully using the five senses. Turn back to Chapter 8 and practice; hear my voice as I walk you through the mindful scan and help you to use your senses. It can be quite scary and then liberating. It really works if you practice it.

Tip: Buy individual-serving packages of cookies. This eliminates the decision about whether or not to eat more.

LOGGING YOUR WAY TO AWARENESS

Phase 2 introduces more choices, offering you the opportunity to decide whether to snack at midmorning or in the late evening. You will decide this by using your newfound hunger/fullness cues. Keep in mind that if you cannot feel these sensations or perhaps fear trusting your gut instinct, have the snack at midmorning. As we discussed in Chapter 2, we know that early eating is associated with greater weight loss. In due time, you will feel more "body aware" and be ready to make more informed choices. But even if you identified with the constant hunger that results from leptin resistance, don't worry. The Body Clock Diet meal structure is designed to keep your body well-fueled but not overfilled even if you misjudge your fullness a bit. Eventually, you will become an expert at recognizing a fullness level of 7 on a scale of 1 to 10 to cue yourself to stop eating. Phase 2's daily logging will help you practice gauging your level of hunger and fullness.

Bear in mind that your daily structure flows with your 24-hour master clock. Continue to rise with the sunshine and get into bed on the earlier side. No late nights out and no eating in the middle of the night. This means no drinking with late-night pizza binges. If you want pizza, eat it for lunch or dinner. If you want alcohol, Phase 2 offers the option of reintroducing a bit of vino.

GUIDELINES FOR PHASE 2

YOUR WATER: Your body is about 65 percent water. Increase your water consumption by 1 cup more per day each week until you're drinking 9 to 11 cups daily. Of course, continue your morning mug of warm water to stimulate peristalsis, the movement of food and waste through your digestive system.

YOUR WINE: Believe it or not, habitual nourishment for a Body Clock lifestyle can include wine in small amounts. But don't get too excited. One glass a day is associated with heart health, but we do not recommend this. If you normally drink wine, you may choose to reintroduce one glass of wine per week for days 15 through 30. If you choose to drink, you must drink on a full stomach, or at least with your dinner meal. Don't forget that alcohol disrupts circadian rhythm and digestion and it impairs judgment around food choices.

YOUR COFFEE: The Body Clock Diet has timed your coffee for 9:00 a.m. consumption. To prevent an exaggerated spike in cortisol and likely weight gain, continue to drink your coffee at about 9:00 a.m., when cortisol is likely falling.

YOUR SUGAR: If you want sugar in your coffee, use sugar, as in sucrose. Beware that many "natural" sugar substitutes actually have added erythritol and maltodextrin. If you want to use stevia, buy 100 percent pure stevia. Read the ingredients to ensure that it is truly 100 percent stevia.

6:00 a.m.—Snooze

You know the drill: Sleep longer if you can. If you wake early, that's great, because you're likely in sync with the diurnal clock known as light and dark. Get up and start your day. You may adjust the schedule accordingly. If you're forced to get up early and still feel tired, try going to bed earlier. Also, if you're the kind of girl who dashes out the door, take some mindful breaths on your way to the office and just be mindful of what you're doing even while you're walking.

7:00 a.m.—No Need for the Alarm

Lucky you, if you got to sleep in. Give yourself and/or your partner a morning hug and set an intention for the day. If your breakfast is quinoa, go ahead and make that first while sipping your mug of hot water. Then shower and eat. Remember to pack a toothbrush and toothpaste for your shoulder bag.

8:00 a.m.—Eat to the Beat

Keep your body clock in rhythm. Grab your mindful meal log and turn inward. Rate your level of hunger, jot down your thoughts and feelings, and then eat. Remember to log after your meal as well.

Phase 2 Breakfasts

- **MAKE ME:** Apple-Cinnamon Quinoa Breakfast Bowl (page 148)

- **TIME CRUNCH:** Easy Eggs Antigua (page 147)

- **EAT IN OR OUT:** Greek yogurt with a pack of oatmeal. This option is easily purchased on the go at your local coffee shop and very likely your local pharmacy. You can also purchase oatmeal from Starbucks or a place like Pret A Manger. I really love Pret's multigrain hot cereal. When eating out, there are many distractions, so focus on the task at hand: checking in with your internal cues.

9:00 a.m.—Coffee Break

Enjoy a coffee of your choice with a milk of your choice. If you're trying to lower your cortisol and lose weight, refrain from using added sugars. This means limiting flavored syrups, toppings, and even sugar-free substitutes. The spike in glucose, insulin, and cortisol isn't worth it. As far as the sugar substitutes go, research shows there's an association between diet drinks and obesity. It's just an association, but additional research suggests the artificial sugar confuses the mind-body biological processes. The Body Clock Diet is about removing body confusion, not adding more.

10:00 a.m.—Zen Me a Snack!

Get Zen and check in with your internal sensations of hunger and fullness. Decide if you want to have your midmorning snack. If you relate to a number 5 on the scale, you can likely wait. If you question or even fear your ability to understand the internal sensations, by all means have the snack. There is no right or wrong. As time goes on, you will begin to develop more self-trust.

Zen Snacks (choose one)

- 1 small piece of fruit and 16 almonds

- 1 Clif Kid Z bar (for kids but gals can eat them too)

- 1 small piece of fruit and 1 or 2 mini Babybel cheeses

12:00 Noon—Lunch

Lunch is a must. Phase 2 offers the perfect practical experience to eat all foods by introducing all foods.

- **MAKE ME:** Roasted Veggies with Chicken Sausage or tofu (page 152)

- **TIME CRUNCH:** Tuna-Filled Pita with a Side of Oreos (page 154; who doesn't like a glass of milk with cookies?)

- **EAT IN OR OUT:** Granny Smith Goat Cheese Sandwich (page 151) with an individual bag of natural popcorn

- **COOKIE CRUSH:** This is the time to flip back to Chapter 8 and review how to eat an Oreo. If you prefer, by all means have chips or whatever you love. The food itself is not that important; rather, the experience is. You must give yourself permission. The *Women's Health* Body Clock Diet gives you permission to eat this lunch side. Yes, it is a side to your sandwich. You have chosen to eat all foods, and you're learning how. Savor, relish, and speak kind words to yourself. You can eat all foods some of the time—aka moderation.

3:30 p.m.—Like Clockwork

Prevent temptation during this cortisol downgrade.

First, make your entry in the Body Clock log. We encourage you to do this before you eat and/or drink anything. Take a Dirgha breath and check in. Mindfully eat your snack using your five senses and then move your body. Make the effort to either walk around the office or the house or outside after meals. Not only will it help to bring awareness to your body, but research correlates walking after meals with decreased blood glucose, insulin, cortisol, and triglycerides and even with weight loss.

Zen Snacks (choose one)

- 1 cup whole wheat pretzels with 100-calorie pack of Wholly Guacamole or about 4 tablespoons of guacamole

- 1 fat-free fruit-flavored Greek yogurt

- 4 ounces cottage cheese with 1 cup berries

6:00 p.m.—Mindfulness Exercise

Hopefully you're home, and if not, try to get at least 5 minutes to yourself. My preference is longer. This is the time to review your *Women's Health* Body Clock logs and notice any patterns or trends that may be helpful or hurtful. Use this time to observe tension in your mind and body. Diffuse this stress with the Cortisol Crushers. After this reset, get ready for your dining experience.

6:30 p.m.—Dinner

This is not any ordinary dinner. This is your mindful connection to food. Set the table with candles, new dishes, or even a new place mat. Eat in a place where you feel comfortable and relaxed. These little things affect how satisfied you are with your meal. The key to portion management when honoring your needs is to be sated and satisfied. Aim to complete your meal at full, not stuffed.

- **MAKE ME:** Garlicky Shrimp with Spaghetti Squash and Spinach (page 158)

- **TIME CRUNCH:** Orecchiette with Pesto and Sausage (page 155)

- **EAT IN OR OUT:** BBQ Chicken with Sweet Potato and Roasted Broccoli (page 156)

8:00 p.m.—Project Self

This is your time to "sharpen the saw." Some nights it will be an art project, journaling, or reading, while other nights it will be exercising. Just be you. Project Self is the act of self-care through mindfulness before and after dinner and movement or skills/distractions after dinner. If you are not moving, refer to the comfort card. The goals of Project Self are to banish cortisol cravings, hedonic hunger, behavioral eating, and emotional eating. Go ahead; counter the fall in cortisol by going to the gym when you would otherwise be home watching TV and grazing on snacks.

10:30 p.m.—Meditation My Way

Try meditating for just 1 minute before bed. This is Mindfulness 101. There are no expectations. You don't need to sit like Buddha or even quiet your mind. You can do the four-square breathing from yoga teacher Jen G. You can do the Dirgha breath or you can just sit for 1 minute and listen to the sounds around you or even the lyrics of your music. This is the no-judgment zone!

Sleep well! Rest, and repeat this daily structure for the next 2 weeks. Each day take note of our recommended awareness. Refer to Chapters 7 and 8 as needed. Switch up your meals each day so you get to find your favorites. Notice which meals and movements energize you and which you would prefer to skip.

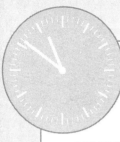

PHASE 2 SAMPLE MINDFUL MEAL LOG

MORNING CHECK-IN:

Wake-Up Time	Hours Slept	Quality of Sleep	Feelings, Thoughts, Behaviors
	8hrs	Great sleep	

Type of Hunger	Feelings, Thoughts, Behaviors Before	Food Eaten	Feelings, Thoughts, Behaviors After

BREAKFAST
Time: 8 a.m.

Emotional Behavioral (Physical)	Hungry and happy Can't wait to try new recipes.	Apple-Cinnamon Quinoa Breakfast Bowl (page 148)	Satiated and satisfied

Tools Used: Four-square breathing before meal

Hunger/Fullness Before Meal: 1 2 ③ 4 5 6 7 8 9 10   Hunger/Fullness After Meal: 1 2 3 4 5 6 ⑦ 8 9 10

MIDMORNING SNACK
Time: 10:30 a.m.

Emotional Behavioral (Physical)	Not necc. ready for meal but nervous to try hunger fullness cues. Think I will try it on another day, especially since we are having a lunch meeting. Maybe tomorrow I will skip snack and have an earlier lunch.	Clif Bar	Loved it. So happy to have something I didn't have to prepare. Perfect size.

Tools Used: Logging

Hunger/Fullness Before Meal: 1 2 ③ 4 5 6 7 8 9 10   Hunger/Fullness After Meal: 1 2 3 4 5 6 ⑦ 8 9 10

LUNCH
Time: 2 p.m.

Emotional (Behavioral) (Physical)	Ready to eat but also eating now because of lunch meeting. Feel okay bringing my own meal into the meeting. Will do Oreo lunch tomorrow. So excited for this.	Roasted Veggies with Chicken Sausage (page 152)	OMG! This meal is so filling I could probably have stopped a few bites early, but I wasn't paying attention to my cues. Was in the meeting and lost focus.

Tools Used: Meal structure

Hunger/Fullness Before Meal: 1 2 ③ 4 5 6 7 8 9 10   Hunger/Fullness After Meal: 1 2 3 4 5 6 7 ⑧ 9 10

Type of Hunger	Feelings, Thoughts, Behaviors Before	Food Eaten	Feelings, Thoughts, Behaviors After

TEMPTATION TIME

Time: 4:30 p.m.

(Emotional) Behavioral (Physical)	Happy to eat and break from work. Feel irritated by coworker but I am truly hungry.	Greek yogurt	Very cool to take time for me and actually practice the body scan Laura shared with us. Individual Greek yogurt is sweet enough but not enough to make me start craving sweets.

Tools Used: Dirgha breath and body scan

Hunger/Fullness Before Meal: 1 2 ③ 4 5 6 7 8 9 10   Hunger/Fullness After Meal: 1 2 3 4 5 6 ⑦ 8 9 10

MINDFULNESS EXERCISE

Tools Used:
Logging and self-care by allowing myself to have downtime. Feel energized now that I stopped going going.

Feelings, Thoughts, Behaviors:
Used this time to read the Five Pillars, check over my logs, and get dinner ready.

DINNER

Time: 6:30–6:48 p.m.

Emotional Behavioral (Physical)	Wonder if this meal will fill me. It was super easy to make. Not sure if I will do physical activity tonight or paint.	Garlicky Shrimp with Spaghetti Squash and Spinach (page 158)	Just the right size for me and not stuffed, so I think I will try the movement piece tonight.

Tools Used: Meal structure, logging, self-care

Hunger/Fullness Before Meal: 1 2 ③ 4 5 6 7 8 9 10   Hunger/Fullness After Meal: 1 2 3 4 5 6 7 ⑧ 9 10

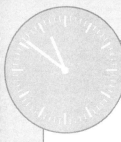

PHASE 2
MINDFUL MEAL LOG

MORNING CHECK-IN:

Wake-Up Time	Hours Slept	Quality of Sleep	Feelings, Thoughts, Behaviors

Type of Hunger	Feelings, Thoughts, Behaviors Before	Food Eaten	Feelings, Thoughts, Behaviors After
BREAKFAST			Time:
Emotional Behavioral Physical			
Tools Used:			
Hunger/Fullness Before Meal: 1 2 3 4 5 6 7 8 9 10		Hunger/Fullness After Meal: 1 2 3 4 5 6 7 8 9 10	
MIDMORNING SNACK			Time:
Emotional Behavioral Physical			
Tools Used:			
Hunger/Fullness Before Meal: 1 2 3 4 5 6 7 8 9 10		Hunger/Fullness After Meal: 1 2 3 4 5 6 7 8 9 10	
LUNCH			Time:
Emotional Behavioral Physical			
Tools Used:			
Hunger/Fullness Before Meal: 1 2 3 4 5 6 7 8 9 10		Hunger/Fullness After Meal: 1 2 3 4 5 6 7 8 9 10	

* Make copies of these log pages.

Type of Hunger	Feelings, Thoughts, Behaviors Before	Food Eaten	Feelings, Thoughts, Behaviors After

TEMPTATION TIME   Time:

Emotional Behavioral Physical			

Tools Used:

Hunger/Fullness Before Meal: 1 2 3 4 5 6 7 8 9 10   Hunger/Fullness After Meal: 1 2 3 4 5 6 7 8 9 10

MINDFULNESS EXERCISE

Tools Used:	Feelings, Thoughts, Behaviors:

DINNER   Time:

Emotional Behavioral Physical			

Tools Used:

Hunger/Fullness Before Meal: 1 2 3 4 5 6 7 8 9 10   Hunger/Fullness After Meal: 1 2 3 4 5 6 7 8 9 10

CHAPTER
10

Skill Builder: Mindfulness, Meditation, and Compassion

PRACTICAL STRATEGIES FOR CRUSHING THE CORTISOL MONSTER

By now I hope you're convinced that reducing stress in your life is critically important for stabilizing and maintaining your body clock and thereby losing weight. When stress happens, your body's cells react with a surge of adrenaline and the stress hormone cortisol. Cortisol tells your body to replenish energy, so you crave energy-dense foods, and it also encourages your body to store fat. It's a double whammy to be avoided.

But in our modern world, stress is unavoidable. Since stress isn't going to evaporate anytime soon, you need to learn effective ways to ease stress or reduce its damaging effects on your body. This skills chapter will show you how to use self-compassion, mindfulness, and meditation to decrease cortisol and increase feel-good chemicals such as oxytocin that soothe and calm.

MINDFULNESS AND SELF-COMPASSION

You have already been practicing mindfulness by writing down your thoughts and feelings in your Body Clock Diet mindful meal log. The exercise forces you to become more aware of when and why you're eating, which is an important step in identifying emotional hunger and behavioral hunger and ultimately reducing "mindless" calorie consumption. Mindfulness is an effective tool against compulsive habits like binge eating because it interrupts automatic behaviors. It enables you to see and understand your actions without judging them to short-circuit the process that connects stress with comfort eating. In a study funded by the National Institutes of Health, researchers tracked the eating patterns of 140 binge eaters and found that using mindfulness-based interventions reduced bingeing episodes from four times to only once per week.

Practicing mindfulness also can help you become better at another key stress buster: self-compassion. What often happens when you eat an extra slice of chocolate cake or you notice a roll of fat bulging out of your shirt as you pass by a mirror? Many women default to judging themselves harshly and criticizing themselves. It's a self-inflicted attack that becomes a real threat. The body automatically acts to defend itself against the attack by releasing excess cortisol. Researchers studying these processes have concluded that criticism and shame are among the most powerful triggers of the cortisol stress response. And as you already know, cortisol can upset your body clock. This is the very reason why you need to be kind to yourself.

Kristin Neff, PhD, a self-compassion researcher and author, says there are three core components to learning self-compassion: self-kindness, common humanity, and mindfulness. Here's how to put them into practice.

1. **Treat yourself with kindness.** Here's a terrific way to be kind to yourself that I learned from one of my clients: When you notice self-criticism creeping in, talk to yourself (in your internal dialogue) the same way you would speak to a child—compassionately.

2. **Identify how you're similar to others.** Recognize that you aren't the only one in this world who is suffering. Suffering and personal inadequacy are part of

the human experience. As Neff says, "To be human is to be imperfect." This is the one commonality we all share.

3. **Live in the present moment.** By being mindful of our negative emotions and thoughts we can observe them with openness and clarity and avoid blowing them out of proportion.

DIY: AN EASY MEDITATION EXERCISE

Now that you're readying yourself to work your way through Phase 3, you're primed for some expert advice on meditation. My dear friend and colleague Adrienne Glasser is an experiential psychotherapist in New York City who founded Experience Wellness Group. The group combines experiential methods, the creative arts, and meditation in a therapy called Active Mindfulness. She shares some effective techniques to help increase body awareness in the simple beginner meditation below. Find a quiet space and give it a try.

Preparation

- Find a comfortable seat that allows you to feel strong but also has a sense of softness or gentleness.

- If you're on the floor, make sure your hips are above your knees. If you're in a chair, make sure you're in an upright position that isn't stiff.

- Allow your shoulders to drop and softly let your arms fall to your sides.

- Gently place your hands on your midthighs or in your lap.

- You can choose to close your eyes, keep them open and gaze about 3 to 4 feet in front of you, or look at these words on the paper as you practice.

Check-In (a few moments)

In these few moments, observe the quality of your mind. Is it fast? Slow? Hazy? What is the temperature of the mind in this moment? Notice these qualities as if you're looking at the ocean, accepting any waves that come.

Intention (a few moments)

Set an intention of observing a sensation in the body and distinguishing it from thoughts about the body. This distinction affords you greater clarity to more intimately know your body and its needs.

Notice the Breath (a few moments)

See where you notice the breath the most in this moment. Is it in your chest, rising and falling? Your nostrils? Your belly? This point where you notice the breath can be like a lighthouse on the ocean, a beacon you can come back to anytime you become lost.

Notice Sensations around the Breath (a few minutes)

Notice what sensations you feel in your body. These sensations are like the different qualities of water in the ocean. Notice whether the sensations make your body want to move or be still. If organic movement starts, just allow this to happen and then let it pass.

You can label sensations as pleasant, unpleasant, or neutral.

Feel free to use your own one-word sensation labels describing the quality of sensation, such as hot, cold, tight, soft, numb, etc. Always come back to the breath as the sturdy lighthouse that accepts all without wavering.

Observe Thoughts Passing (a few minutes)

- Envision thoughts that may come in as if they're boats on the ocean. Notice how thoughts about the body are different from sensation felt in the body. Allow the boats of thought to freely float through the waves of sensations. If a boat of thought grabs your attention, perhaps see what message it wants you to hear and then allow it to pass.

- Know you can always come back to the lighthouse of the breath if you get lost at sea.

- Continue to label the sensations in the body simply, distinguishing these simple observations from thought: pleasant, unpleasant, neutral . . .

- Repeat this observation of sensation, thoughts floating, then back to breath.

Gratitude (a few moments)

Honor your higher sense of knowing, which helped you throughout this practice.

Thank yourself for your efforts, knowing that the merit of your practice will benefit your body and those you love.

CHAPTER
11

Phase 3: Rock Your Clock

DAYS 31 TO 45: ADDING MORE FLEXIBILITY TO A LIFE OF QUIET STRENGTH AND CONTROL

By now, the fifth week of your Body Clock Diet Program, you should start to see and feel significant differences in your body. Your jeans are looser. Your belly is tighter. You can manage stress much more effectively thanks to the tools and the exercise programs.

I hope you're seeing this and recognizing that it's all due to simplifying your life, understanding the benefits of positive nutrition, and establishing patterns of eating and sleeping that remove opportunities to lose mindfulness and overeat.

Again, let's review those steps that should be rote by the start of Phase 3.

1. You're starting every morning with a mug of warm water. It's a habitual beginning to the day and sends a powerful message to your brain that it's going to be one of healthy and mindful living.

2. You're staying off the scale. Instead you're focused on eating enough food and calories to maintain your high metabolism and the muscle mass you've built through strength training.

3. You're eating all foods, even enjoying cookies like you never have before.

4. One glass of wine is enough for you. You savor it.

5. Your cravings have vanished and the meal structure has allowed you to listen to your internal cues driving hunger and fullness.

6. Breathing techniques, Cortisol Crushers, the comfort card, and other tools have replaced cravings and automatic behaviors. The 3:00 to 4:00 p.m. time slot is now dedicated to a planned snack and a brief walk to increase alertness naturally.

7. The structure of your sleep is now routine and habitual, synchronized to honor your body clock and Earth's rotation.

8. You're becoming adept at internal self-awareness to connect with hunger/ fullness cues as well as a greater understanding of how the mind-body and even belly-brain act as one.

9. You understand how cortisol, the stress hormone, can knock your clock off track and that you must decrease your chronic stress to rock with your clock for life.

You're doing great! Now, over the final 14 days, you'll become more flexible with your meal structure, which will challenge you to adapt and grow stronger, more self-compassionate, and smarter, leading to a Body Clock lifestyle.

BEND TO BECOME STRONGER

"The tree that bends to the winds will last much longer
than its stiff-limbed neighbor."
—Edward J. Lavin, SJ, in *Life Meditations*

The quote above is one of my favorites, and I feel it is so appropriate for Phase 3 of the Body Clock Diet, because this final phase is the one you'll use for life to maintain the great strides you will have made over the past 6 weeks.

Have you ever spent time in a forest during a rain-and-wind storm or at least watched hurricane-force winds batter a tropical coast? Perhaps you've noticed that some trees—usually the stiff-limbed, more mature ones—don't bend very much against the wind. They try to fight the wind, withstand its relentless power, and ultimately crack or break. Now focus on the more nimble, younger trees whose narrow green trunks bend and sway but stay intact.

I want you to be like a young tree that bends as you embark on Phase 3 and beyond. You will eat with much more flexibility during the next 14 days; all foods still fit, but now you'll eat everyday foods (fresh, whole foods containing a mix of the three macronutrients) the majority of the time and sometimes foods (low-nutrition foods) about a quarter of the time. You will use the tools of meditation, mindfulness, and self-compassion, and you will become more body aware.

Increase your stress tolerance with yoga and do more advanced strength-training and cardio exercises to boost your metabolism. You will learn to defeat self-criticism and honor your mind-body by connecting them ever more organically to your biological rhythms. Here are your four ways to be clock wise during Phase 3.

GUIDELINES FOR PHASE 3

YOUR WATER: Increase your water consumption by 1 cup more per day each week until you achieve 9 to 11 cups daily. Remember to include your morning mug of warm-to-hot water to awaken your gut.

YOUR WINE: Red, white, or rosé. You may choose to include two glasses of wine per week for days 31 through 45. If you choose to drink, be sure to have your first glass of alcohol with or after your meal. Drink it slowly and mindfully. Notice the bouquet, the legs, and the mouthfeel. Notice which wines you prefer with different foods. Notice the next morning if the alcohol affects your digestion, hunger sensations, or hydration status. Alcohol disrupts circadian rhythm and digestion and impairs judgment around food choices.

YOUR COMPASSION: Over the next 2 weeks, you will be intent on increasing self-compassion as discussed in Chapter 10. You will notice that your new Body Clock Mindful Meals Log includes an additional column to the right: "Reframe with Kindness." For every self-criticism and every negative thought, you can counter it in the kindness column. This will help to create the automatic compassionate thought, feeling, or behavior rather than self-sabotage or self-criticism.

YOUR CUDDLE: Oxytocin is a natural hormone known as the "hug hormone" and the "cuddle chemical" because our pituitary gland at the base of the brain secretes it when we kiss or hug someone we love. It's a powerful neurotransmitter that combats stress and anxiety. That's why it's so useful for the Body Clock Diet. Use soft touch and hugs with a loved one or even sweet thoughts about someone special to increase this feel-good hormone.

7:00 a.m.—Wake-Up Time

Hopefully, waking is easier in weeks 5 and 6. Take advantage of this increase in cortisol and get yourself ready. Start by getting a little TLC from your partner, your pet, and yourself! Talk kindly to yourself. Tell yourself, *"I am okay. I am healthy."* If you have the time, meditate. Use Adrienne Glasser's meditation guide. Start with 1 minute and increase by 1 minute every day until you achieve 20 minutes. The goal is to just take time to be silent and be aware of your sensations.

8:00 a.m.—Breakfast

Boost the morning with one of these three options.

- **MAKE ME:** Simple Mediterranean Breakfast (page 160) with Israeli Salad (page 161). Break the fast with fresh veggies, olive oil, eggs, and of course, some feta!

- **TIME CRUNCH:** Vanilla Chia Pudding with Berries (page 163). Make this the night before or as soon as you wake up. It can set while you dress and be ready to eat in just 15 minutes. This is a protein- and fat-packed recipe.

- **EAT IN OR OUT:** Protein-Packed Toast (page 164). Smear on hummus and cucumbers for the best crunch. This is also an easy choice for on the go. Just ask the deli to make this specific open-faced sandwich. This is your third breakfast option to choose while in or out of your own kitchen. Eating all foods and being healthy was never so easy.

9:00 a.m.—Coffee Mate

Check in with yourself. If you want to increase alertness, grab a cup of joe. You can add milk for calcium.

10:00 a.m.—Midmorning Mindfulness

From this day forward, associate 10:00 a.m. with your morning check-in. Take a few moments to do a body scan from Chapter 8, take a Dirgha breath, and recognize your level of hunger or fullness. Decide whether you want to snack now or later. You are a competent eater. You can choose. Go ahead and eat mindfully for physical hunger. If it's a rocky morning and you choose to eat for emotional or behavioral hunger, make the decision and don't look back. Regrets are not needed in your new lifestyle. There is no guilt; rather there are choices and consequences.

Soul Snacks

Choose from one of the three options below.

- 4 ounces 100% juice with ¼ cup roasted nuts

- 3 pieces no-sugar-added dried fruit and 4 ounces cottage cheese

- ¼ cup granola with ½ cup full-fat Greek yogurt

12:00 Noon—Lunch

Choose from and then log one of your new recipes.

- **MAKE ME:** Make Me Greek Salad Wrap (page 165)

- **TIME CRUNCH:** Veggie Burger with a Side of Fruit and "Sometimes Food" (page 166)

- **EAT IN OR OUT:** Panera Flatbread or a Tomato-Basil-Mozzarella Sandwich with Tomato Soup (page 167)

3:30 p.m.—Tame Temptation Time

It's likely this is an easy time of day for you by weeks 5 and 6. Don't get uppity, get real. Stick to this snack time no matter what. Do not skip! It's crucial to eat at this time, when cortisol is crashing and fatigue is starting to set in.

Snack Pack

Choose one of three snacks.

- Banana and 1 heaping tablespoon of natural nut butter

- Gluten-free muffin with a glass of milk (the gluten-free muffins you buy from the freezer section are typically smaller than deli muffins and more filling; try Glutino muffins)

- Black bean chips and guacamole (try Better Way Chips and Wholly Guacamole Single Packs)

When snacking is over, make time for movement. Climb the stairs at the office or practice improving stress tolerance with the yoga moves from Chapter 13 for 5 to 10 minutes. You can also take this time to reflect on your observations when reviewing your Mindful Meal Log.

5:30 p.m.—Pre-Exercise Snack

Yes, we're throwing you a curveball. You're going to learn in the next 2 weeks how to function in case you need to exercise before coming home to eat dinner. This means eat your second or perhaps third snack at 5:30 before hitting the gym or the spin studio or going for a walk. It's okay if this snack is pure carbohydrate, as your body will quickly lower your blood sugar once you start to move. This is also the ideal snack and exercise time if you have difficulty falling asleep or your sleep quality is a problem.

Quick Fix

Choose one of three snacks.

- 1 to 2 cups fresh-cut fruit such as orange, pineapple, or pear

- 1 Clif Kid Z bar

- 1 cup raw cauliflower and carrots with 2 tablespoons honey-mustard dressing

6:00 p.m.—Exercise or Project Self

Now that you're charged and ready, you're getting tested. That's right—before the clock strikes, we're seeing if you can be flexible yet structured. Whether you exercise at 9:30 a.m. or 8:30 p.m., the most important thing to do is stay consistent with behaviors, minimize your stress levels, and boost positive compassion. So this week, try exercising before dinner. Listen inward to see which rhythm meshes best with you. If this is a night off from movement, cook one of the Make Me dinners, since they take a few more minutes to prepare than the others. In addition, use this time to log, to do a mindful body scan, and to cuddle up.

8:00 p.m.—Dinner

Did you ever think someone would say eat at 8:00 p.m.? Probably not. Since this is a lifestyle, and late dinners are a reality for many, it's important to address. Research shows that lunch needs to be eaten before 3:00 p.m., but there's no mention of dinnertime. These meals are balanced and portioned. Be realistic and think long-term. Do what you can and leave the rest to meditation. That's the whole point of being flexible and self-compassionate.

Be mindful of logging hunger/fullness and using the five senses when you dine. Set a pretty table, light some candles, or even play music while you cook. Be in the moment. Be sure you're eating enough but not stuffing yourself. You are your portion maker. Some days you may need more food, and some days you may need less food. Just bear in mind the structure and the concept of mixed meals with carbohydrates, proteins, and fat. Aim for 75 percent everyday foods and 25 percent sometimes foods.

- **MAKE ME:** Pasta and Sautéed Brussels Sprouts with Pine Nuts and Parmesan (page 170)

- **TIME CRUNCH:** Fast Chicken Fajitas (page 169)

- **EAT IN OR OUT:** Simply Satisfying Salmon with Garlicky Haricots Verts (page 168)

9:00 p.m.—Mindfulness and Meditation

Turn inward before bed. This is a good time to do an art project, lengthen your chosen mindfulness activity, or use the beginner's easy meditation on page 113. Start with 1 minute and add 1 minute each night until you achieve 20 minutes.

10:00 p.m.—Silent Night

It's time to rest and digest, cuddle your cortisol down, and be silent.

BEYOND PHASE 3: THE BODY CLOCK DIET LIFESTYLE

You have achieved 45 days of self-care, mindfulness, and movement. You're living and breathing in kindness. You know how to maintain your metabolism, decrease stress, and tick to the tune of your circadian rhythm. You have a bucket of tools and recipes to keep your body clock in sync.

Going forward, use the Phase 3 Body Clock Mindful Meal Log and journal every 3 days to ensure you always stay aware of your needs and hungers. If you're eating out, remember to practice mindful eating. Restaurant meals are typically larger and have more calories. Be alert in social situations and especially when drinking alcohol. Observe how you feel when you drink and how it affects you the following day.

Maintain your meal structure. Never skip breakfast and eat an earlier lunch. Use your meal structure to ensure you eat three meals daily and one to three planned snacks pending your hunger. If you feel as if you're losing focus, simply pull out this book and choose one of the phases to resume. Likely Phase 2 or Phase 3 will be sufficient to reground and reset the body clock. I encourage you to use the phases, especially the meal structure, when returning from vacation, overseas travel, or a few stressful weeks.

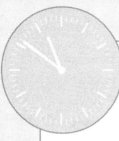

PHASE 3 SAMPLE MINDFUL MEAL LOG

MORNING CHECK-IN:

Wake-Up Time	Hours Slept	Feelings, Thoughts, Behaviors	Food Eaten	GI Symptom If Any	Reframe with Kindness and Note Tool Used
7:45 a.m.	9hrs	I slept one hour longer than I wanted to. Ugh, now I am going to be late.	Mug water	Bowel movement	You need not be perfect. Think of it this way, you got the right amount of sleep.

Feelings, Thoughts, Behaviors Before	Food Eaten	Feelings, Thoughts, Behaviors After	Reframe with Kindness and Note Tool Used
BREAKFAST			**Time:** 8 a.m.
Think hungry but rushing as woke up late so hard to tune in. Will eat because I know I should.	Vanilla Chia Pudding with Berries (page 163)	Thank goodness I made this last night.	Remember to take a breath and read Pillars at work.
GI Symptom:			
Hunger/Fullness Before Meal: 1 2 ③ 4 5 6 7 8 9 10		Hunger/Fullness After Meal: 1 2 3 4 5 6 ⑦ 8 9 10	
MIDMORNING SNACK			**Time:** 11:00 a.m.
Not hungry but did check in. Choosing to not have snack.			Flexibility with structure is my mantra.
GI Symptom:			
Hunger/Fullness Before Meal: 1 2 3 4 ⑤ 6 7 8 9 10		Hunger/Fullness After Meal: 1 2 3 4 5 6 7 8 9 10	
LUNCH			**Time:** 12:15 p.m.
Forgot lunch will step out for Panera sandwich.	Flatbread and small veggie soup	Thank goodness there are options to eat out. Got the soup as knew I would need more food today.	Go back to the office and take a few minutes to do the Dirgha breath and use one of my Cortisol Crushers.
GI Symptom: Stomach feels slightly bloated. Could it be the fiber in the bread, the liquid from the soup, or eating too quickly?			
Hunger/Fullness Before Meal: 1 2 ③ 4 5 6 7 8 9 10		Hunger/Fullness After Meal: 1 2 3 4 5 6 ⑦ 8 9 10	

Feelings, Thoughts, Behaviors Before	Food Eaten	Feelings, Thoughts, Behaviors After	Reframe with Kindness and Note Tool Used

TAME TEMPTATION
Time: 3 p.m.

Day been going too fast. I am intentionaly carving out time to do some meditation before my snack.	Banana and PB	Feel better and calm	You did an awesome job with self-care and compassion. Used meditation.

GI Symptom:

Hunger/Fullness Before Meal: 1 2 ③ 4 5 6 7 8 9 10   Hunger/Fullness After Meal: 1 2 3 4 5 6 ⑦ 8 9 10

PRE-EXERCISE SNACK
Time: 5 p.m.

Eating now as exercising before dinner and know I will not last without a snack.	Pear	Fine	Mindful eating

GI Symptom:

Hunger/Fullness Before Meal: 1 2 3 4 ⑤ 6 7 8 9 10   Hunger/Fullness After Meal: 1 2 3 4 5 6 ⑦ 8 9 10

DINNER
Time: 7:30 p.m.

Rocking to my clock!	Simply Satisfying Salmon with Garlicky Haricots Verts (page 168)	Love, love, love this dish	Making dinner for myself feels so good.

GI Symptom:

Hunger/Fullness Before Meal: 1 ② ③ 4 5 6 7 8 9 10   Hunger/Fullness After Meal: 1 2 3 4 5 6 ⑦ ⑧ 9 10

MIND AND MEDITATION
Time: 9:30 p.m.

Tools Used:	Feelings, Thoughts, Behaviors:
Read my Pillars. Completed my log and meditated for 10 minutes.	I don't need to perfect meditation. Humans are imperfect.

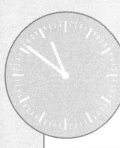

PHASE 3
MINDFUL MEAL LOG

MORNING CHECK-IN:

Wake-Up Time	Hours Slept	Feelings, Thoughts, Behaviors	Food Eaten	GI Symptom If Any	Reframe with Kindness and Note Tool Used

Feelings, Thoughts, Behaviors Before	Food Eaten	Feelings, Thoughts, Behaviors After	Reframe with Kindness and Note Tool Used
BREAKFAST			Time:

GI Symptom:

Hunger/Fullness Before Meal: 1 2 3 4 5 6 7 8 9 10   Hunger/Fullness After Meal: 1 2 3 4 5 6 7 8 9 10

MIDMORNING SNACK			Time:

GI Symptom:

Hunger/Fullness Before Meal: 1 2 3 4 5 6 7 8 9 10   Hunger/Fullness After Meal: 1 2 3 4 5 6 7 8 9 10

LUNCH			Time:

GI Symptom:

Hunger/Fullness Before Meal: 1 2 3 4 5 6 7 8 9 10   Hunger/Fullness After Meal: 1 2 3 4 5 6 7 8 9 10

* Make copies of these log pages.

Feelings, Thoughts, Behaviors Before	Food Eaten	Feelings, Thoughts, Behaviors After	Reframe with Kindness and Note Tool Used
TAME TEMPTATION			Time:
GI Symptom:			
Hunger/Fullness Before Meal: 1 2 3 4 5 6 7 8 9 10		Hunger/Fullness After Meal: 1 2 3 4 5 6 7 8 9 10	
PRE-EXERCISE SNACK			Time:
GI Symptom:			
Hunger/Fullness Before Meal: 1 2 3 4 5 6 7 8 9 10		Hunger/Fullness After Meal: 1 2 3 4 5 6 7 8 9 10	
DINNER			Time:
GI Symptom:			
Hunger/Fullness Before Meal: 1 2 3 4 5 6 7 8 9 10		Hunger/Fullness After Meal: 1 2 3 4 5 6 7 8 9 10	
MIND AND MEDITATION			Time:

CHAPTER
12

The Body Clock
Diet Recipes

DELICIOUS MEALS TO SATISFY
REAL HUNGER . . . IN THE NICK OF TIME!

Now for the tasty part of resetting your internal timer. These are some of my favorite recipes. They're delicious, easy to prepare, and perfect for helping you lose weight naturally without the sabotaging effects of restrictive dieting.

The recipes are organized according to the three phases of the 6-week Body Clock Diet reset program. They're designed to provide a simple structure as you reestablish a rhythm of healthy eating at 2- to 4-hour intervals to avoid blood sugar fluctuations that encourage cravings and trigger bingeing. I recommend these meals as a guideline because I have found that people like to be given some structure when changing lifestyle habits. The recipes on the following pages are organized by phase, but feel free to eat any of the meals in the previous phases as you progress. The ultimate purpose is for you to develop your ideal eating rhythm and portion sizes and eventually bring your own favorite meals into the mix. Delicious, healthy food is one of the great joys of life, and a body in balance is one that feels happy and satisfied without food guilt. Each meal option, whether breakfast, lunch, or dinner, includes a meal that can be made in a jiff, a meal that requires some time and attention, and of course a meal that can be purchased on the go if time is limited.

While I don't advocate calorie counting, I have included calories and other nutrition information at the end of each recipe because knowing what you're consuming is an important part of healthy eating. It's also there to show you the amounts of the important macronutrients (protein, fat, and carbohydrates) that you're getting in each meal. So remember, all foods are okay. No restrictions. Just *mangia!* And let your body clock keep you at a healthy weight.

Game Changers

Staples for Your Pantry

The Hamptons Honey Company Pure Honey with Comb

Stiles Apiaries Honey, 100% Pure

Natural nut butters, with no added oils or sugars—Our favorite? Vermont Peanut Butter Company

BREAKFAST

PHASE 1: Time Crunch

Peanut Butter Overnight Oats

Makes 1 serving

Pile these filling ingredients in an airtight container—like a mason jar—and enjoy an easy, time-saving breakfast in the morning. Make this recipe with your favorite milk, whether it's plant based or from a cow or even a goat.

⅔ cup unsweetened almond milk

¼ teaspoon ground cinnamon

1 teaspoon raw honey

½ cup rolled oats

1 tablespoon warmed natural peanut butter

1 teaspoon chia seeds (optional)

1. In a medium bowl, whisk together the milk, cinnamon, and honey.

2. Stir in the oats and peanut butter until well combined. Add the chia seeds (if using). Pour the mixture into an airtight container such as a mason jar and refrigerate overnight.

3. When ready to eat, stir the oat mixture and enjoy mindfully.

Per serving: 298 calories, 11 g protein, 38 g carbohydrates, 12 g total fat, 2 g saturated fat, 6 g fiber, 123 mg sodium

Sweet!

A ½-teaspoon drizzle of honey has antibacterial properties.

Avocado Toast*

Makes 1 serving

Try this energy-boosting open-faced sandwich made with a ripe avocado and two spoonfuls of Siggi's Icelandic yogurt. You get just enough yogurt to add a punch of protein to make your meal well balanced, aka a "mixed" meal, and filling.

2 slices Ezekiel bread

½ medium Hass avocado

2 tablespoons Siggi's Plain 0% Skyr yogurt

Salt and black pepper to taste

2 teaspoons red-pepper flakes (optional)

2 ounces heirloom tomatoes (optional)

1. Pop the bread slices into the toaster. Meanwhile, in a small bowl, mash the avocado and combine it with the yogurt. Season the mash with salt and pepper and a dash of red-pepper flakes, if using, for a hint of spice.

2. Spread the mixture onto the toast. Top with the tomatoes, if using, and add a touch of salt and pepper to taste.

Per serving: 395 calories, 16 g protein, 41 g carbohydrates, 21 g total fat, 4 g saturated fat, 8.5 g fiber, 161 mg sodium

Recipe adapted from Siggi's Avocado Toast. Used with permission from Siggi's.

Decode Label Lingo

Sprouted grain means whole grains are soaked until they're newly sprouted. This process increases their levels of antioxidants and B vitamins.

Enriched is an alias for refined white flour with a few vitamins thrown in. Skip breads with this on the bag.

Game Changers

High-Protein Yogurts

Siggi's Icelandic-Style Yogurt

Chobani Greek Yogurt

Fage All Natural Greek Strained Yogurt

Whole Grain Breads

Food for Life Ezekiel 4:9 Sprouted Grain Bread

Vermont Bread Company Organic Whole Wheat or Sprouted Grain

Rudi's Organic Bakery Breads

Whole Foods 365 Organic Bread

Avocado

Avocado is a tasty and versatile craving killer that could help you avoid midmorning hunger pangs (and the snack run that goes with them). Recent research published in *Nutrition Journal* found that adding half an avocado to people's meal decreased their desire to eat over the next 3 hours by a whopping 40 percent.

Granola and Greek Yogurt

Makes 1 serving

This carb-rich breakfast is sure to spark your a.m. energy! Plus, KIND granola contains inulin, an added fiber with prebiotics to help your bowels follow your body clock. Note: Increase fiber to your diet gradually; too much can cause bloating and GI upset.

¾ cup granola, such as KIND Healthy Grains Maple Quinoa Clusters with Chia Seeds

¾ cup Greek full-fat yogurt

In a bowl, mix the granola with the yogurt.

Per serving: 483 calories, 24 g protein, 58 g carbohydrates, 18 g total fat, 7.5 g saturated fat, 7 g fiber, 115 mg sodium

Game Changers

Cold Cereals

KIND Healthy Grains Maple Quinoa Clusters with Chia Seeds

Nature's Path Organic Fruit and Nut Granola

Morning Measuring Hack

All cereals are not created equal. Most people portion granola as if it's regular cereal. If you're using a calorie-dense granola like Dorset granola, be mindful of your portion. Start with ¼ to ½ cup granola to see if it both satisfies and satiates you.

LUNCH

PHASE I: Time Crunch

Peanut Butter 'n' Berry Sandwich with Greek Yogurt

Makes 1 serving

If you still aren't sold on the taste of Greek yogurt, try this recipe to ease into its texture and flavor. Pairing yogurt with fruit, or trying a fruit-flavored option, will tame the bold, creamy flavor.

2 tablespoons natural peanut butter

2 slices bread, such as Ezekiel

½ cup sliced strawberries

1 cup full-fat Greek yogurt

1. Spread 1 tablespoon of peanut butter on each slice of bread.

2. Top the open slices with strawberries.

3. Close your sandwich and enjoy with a side of Greek yogurt.

Per serving: 583 calories, 38 g protein, 50 g carbohydrates, 26 g total fat, 9 g saturated fat, 9 g fiber, 267 mg sodium

Superswap: Strawberries Instead of Jelly

Strawberries are loaded with vitamin C and folate. In general, berries are some of the most nutritious fruits.

Salmon over Sweet Potatoes and Baby Spinach

Makes 1 serving

Perfectly cooked salmon is the prettiest shade of pink. And beautiful food is a great way to indulge all your senses, helping you feel fuller and more satisfied with your meals. Plus, omega-3 fatty acids in the salmon help conduct nerve signals and decrease the inflammation in your body.

4 ounces wild-caught salmon

1 small sweet potato (about 4 ounces), chopped

2 cups packed baby spinach

½ cup cherry tomatoes

1–2 tablespoons Body Clock Vinaigrette (page 145)

Gimme an *A*! Gimme a *D*!

You may curse your sweet tooth when the number on the scale creeps higher, but the real culprit could be what you're *not* eating. New data in the *Journal of the American College of Nutrition* shows that overweight adults had lower levels of the critical micronutrient vitamin A—which is linked to regulation of fat cells—than their normal-weight peers. Previous research has shown vitamin D–deficient people are also more likely to gain. Get 90 percent of your recommended daily value (600 IU) of D with a 3.5-ounce serving of salmon; half a cup of carrots or baby spinach should provide all the A you need.

1. Preheat the oven to 350°F. Line two 9″ x 13″ baking sheets with foil.

2. Place the salmon on one of the pans, skin side down. Bake for 10 to
    12 minutes or until opaque on the exterior, and set aside to finish
    cooking outside of the oven. Fish continues to cook even after it's
    removed from the oven; it's better to take it out a little early so it
    doesn't overcook.

3. While the fish is in the oven, microwave the sweet potatoes on high for
    3 minutes. Once they're done in the microwave, transfer the potatoes
    to the second foil-lined baking sheet and lightly coat them with canola
    oil spray or brush them with olive oil.

4. Swap the fish for the sweet potatoes in the oven. Switch the oven to
    broil and broil the potatoes on the upper shelf for 3 to 5 minutes, or
    until they're browned.

5. In a medium bowl, combine the spinach, tomatoes, and sweet pota-
    toes and toss with the vinaigrette. Serve the salmon over the greens.

    Per serving: 481 calories, 25 g protein, 29 g carbohydrates, 29 g total fat,
    4.5 g saturated fat, 6 g fiber, 315 mg sodium

Sunny Bowl: Eggs over Mashed Butternut Squash and Kale

Makes 1 serving

Eggs aren't just for breakfast. This warm, sunny dish is just as soothing to look at as it is nutritious, and with 18 grams of protein, it keeps you feeling full past the dreaded midafternoon lull.

2 cups butternut squash, peeled and chopped to 1–1½″ slices

2 cups kale, washed and cut into 2″ pieces

1 teaspoon olive oil

2 eggs

Salt and black pepper to taste

1. Preheat the oven to 400°F. Lightly coat a 9″ x 13″ baking sheet with canola oil spray. Arrange the squash on the baking sheet in a single layer and spray the top of the squash again with canola oil.

2. Place the squash in the oven and bake it for 40 minutes.

3. Once cooked, remove the squash from the oven and allow it to cool, about 5 minutes. Transfer it to an individual serving bowl and mash it with a fork.

4. In a medium bowl, coat the kale with the olive oil and use your hands to massage the leaves—this trick will help you tenderize this veggie's fibrous leaves. Then heat a medium skillet over medium-low heat and sauté the kale for about 5 minutes, or until tender.

5. Transfer the kale to the bowl atop the butternut squash.

6. Using the same skillet you used for the kale, respray the pan with canola oil and set it on medium-low heat. Crack the eggs into the pan and cook for 5 to 6 minutes, or until the tops of the whites are set but the yolk is runny. With a spatula, carefully remove the eggs from the pan. Place the 2 eggs over the kale and squash. Season with salt and pepper.

Per serving: 358 calories, 18 g protein, 47.5 g carbohydrates, 14 g total fat, 3.5 g saturated fat, 8 g fiber, 192 mg sodium

A MUCH-NEEDED EGGS-PLANATION

Label terminology got you scrambled? Here's how egg options break down.

Brown

Color alone doesn't indicate anything about an egg other than the type of chicken that laid it, and it doesn't have an impact on the flavor or nutritional profile.

Cage-Free

This designation means the eggs were laid by chickens that were not confined to cages. But if you want a guarantee that the birds had outdoor access, look for certified organic, free-range eggs instead.

Grade A

Eggs are graded for quality: AA, A, or B. The difference between grades has to do with the white's texture (grade B is thinner) and the yolk's shape (somewhat flattened in grade B eggs). In general, grades AA and A are best for poaching.

Free-Range

This USDA-regulated term indicates that the laying hens were not caged and were given continuous access to the outdoors and unlimited access to food and fresh water.

Omega-3-Enhanced

Chickens that have had an omega-3 supplement added to their food produce eggs that can have three to five times the amount of the beneficial fatty acids that naturally occur in eggs. This could make them a good option if you don't eat much fish.

Antibiotic-Free

Labels can play fast and loose with this terminology, so it can be difficult to tell what's regulated and what's not. The only guaranteed way to know you're purchasing eggs from chickens that have not been treated with antibiotics is to buy certified organic.

Organic

The green USDA label ensures that the eggs came from hens that have at least some access to the outdoors and are fed a 100 percent organic diet free from antibiotics. But the organic label doesn't protect these birds from controversial practices like beak cutting.

DINNER

PHASE I: Make Me

Spaghetti Squash and Meatballs

Makes 4 servings

The idea of squash as a pasta alternative was definitely new to my big, Italian family. But trust me, digging into a big, juicy bowl of spaghetti squash can be just as satisfying as a big bowl of pasta! Just remember, it still counts as a carb!

1 small spaghetti squash (3 pounds)

6 cups fresh spinach

¾ pound (12 ounces) lean ground turkey

1 egg

1 small yellow onion, diced

2 cloves garlic, minced

¼ cup Italian bread crumbs

2 teaspoons Italian seasoning

1 jar (16 ounces) no-sugar-added tomato sauce

½ cup grated Parmesan cheese

1. Cut the squash in half across the width. Scoop out the seeds and discard.

2. Steam each half of the squash. Place the squash in a microwaveable dish cut side down in 1" of water. Microwave on high for about 7 minutes. Let cool cut side up for about 5 minutes. It should be slightly al dente.

3. Using a fork, scrape out the flesh so it looks like spaghetti. Transfer the strands into a clean bowl and set aside.

4. Rinse the spinach leaves and place in a microwaveable bowl with about 1 tablespoon of water. Cover the bowl with plastic wrap and microwave on high for 1 to 2 minutes, or until wilted.

5. Preheat the oven to 375°F. Coat a 9" x 13" baking sheet generously with canola oil spray.

6. In a large bowl, combine the turkey, egg, onion, garlic, bread crumbs, and Italian seasoning. Form 1″ balls, similar to the size of golf balls, or about 2 ounces each. Arrange the meatballs on the baking sheet and bake for 20 minutes. Flip once and continue to bake for another 20 minutes, or until the meat is no longer pink.

7. When the meatballs are almost done, heat the tomato sauce over low heat in a large saucepan. Add the wilted spinach and stir, cooking for 3 to 5 minutes. Remove the meatballs from the oven and add to the sauce. Cook for another 5 minutes, stirring occasionally while letting the flavors marinate.

8. Serve 3 meatballs with about 2 cups spaghetti squash and about ½ cup sauce. Sprinkle with 2 tablespoons of Parmesan cheese. Feel free to add a side of roasted Brussels sprouts, roasted broccoli, or your favorite vegetable. Refrigerate the leftover meatballs for another meal or freeze for later.

Per serving: 455 calories, 36 g protein, 38 g carbohydrates, 21 g total fat, 10 g saturated fat, 3 g fiber, 965 mg sodium

Game Changer

Tomato Sauce in a Jar

Cucina Antica All Natural Pasta Sauce

Chipotle Pork Tenderloin with Baby Kale Salad

Makes 2 servings

This recipe transforms pork tenderloin into a dish that packs a perfect ratio of nutrients—and balance of sweet and savory flavors—to end your day of healthy eating deliciously. Save the leftover sauce in the refrigerator for later in the week.

½ pound pork tenderloin

Salt and black pepper to taste

Non-GMO canola oil, or olive oil

4 cups packed baby kale

4 tablespoons toasted pine nuts

¼ cup grated Parmesan cheese

1–2 tablespoons Body Clock Vinaigrette (page 145)

½ cup Spicy Chipotle Sauce

Spicy Chipotle Sauce

⅓ cup orange juice

¼ teaspoon extra-virgin olive oil

½ teaspoon dry mustard

¼ cup finely chopped dried apricots

1½ teaspoons minced fresh garlic

¾ cup ketchup

½ chipotle pepper (canned in adobo sauce), chopped

1. **To make the pork:** Preheat the broiler.

2. Season the pork with salt and black pepper and other seasonings of choice.

3. In a medium skillet, sear the pork for about 2 minutes on each side, brushing with canola or olive oil until all sides are browned.

4. Place the pork on a broiler pan in the oven and broil for 3 to 5 minutes, until slightly pink in the center and a thermometer inserted in the center registers 145°F. Remove the pork from the oven and allow it to rest for 5 minutes. Cut it into slices. The pork can be slightly pink in the center.

5. **To make the sauce:** In a small saucepan over low heat, whisk together the orange juice, oil, mustard, apricots, garlic, ketchup, and chipotle pepper. Adjust the orange juice according to your preferred sweetness.

6. Stir constantly for about 5 minutes, reducing the sauce.

7. In a large bowl, combine the kale, pine nuts, cheese, and vinaigrette. Serve immediately, with 4 ounces pork topped with chipotle sauce.

    Per serving: 588 calories, 45 g protein, 42 g carbohydrates, 31 g total fat, 6 g saturated fat, 3.5 g fiber, 1,299 mg sodium

Turkey Chili

Makes 4 servings

Whether you call it goulash or chili, everyone has their own take on the classic stew of hearty beans and seasonings. This is a favorite dish to freeze and then enjoy after a tiring day. It's so satisfying, you'll most definitely not be craving sweets before bed.

2 cloves garlic, pressed and minced

2 tablespoons non-GMO canola oil

1 small yellow onion, chopped

1 pound ground lean turkey, bison, or beef

1 can (15 ounces) no-salt-added chickpeas

1 can (15 ounces) no-salt-added kidney beans

1 jar (25 ounces) no-sugar-added tomato sauce

2 teaspoons dried oregano

2 teaspoons Italian seasoning

2 cups organic frozen corn or mixed peas, corn, and carrots

1. In a large, nonstick sauté pan over medium heat, cook the garlic in the canola oil for 2 to 3 minutes, stirring frequently. When the garlic is fragrant, add the onion and stir for 3 minutes, or until caramelized. Add the protein (turkey, bison, or beef) and brown thoroughly.

2. Mix in the chickpeas, kidney beans, tomato sauce, oregano, and Italian seasoning.

3. Add the frozen veggies last to prevent them from getting soggy. When the veggies are warm and cooked through, the dish is ready to eat.

4. Let cool and portion into four 2-cup servings. Freeze two servings in Pyrex glassware for an easy meal in Phases 2 and 3. Refrigerate the third portion for later in Phase 1. You can eat this meal without a side or pair it with a cup of cooked pasta or a baked potato.

VARIATION: *Top your dish with a dollop of full-fat Greek yogurt or a sprinkle of shredded Cheddar cheese.*

Per serving: 576 calories, 48 g protein, 60 g carbohydrates, 21 g total fat, 4 g saturated fat, 17 g fiber, 470 mg sodium

Body Clock Vinaigrette

Makes 16 servings, 1 tablespoon each

Amp up your salad with olive oil–based dressings! Add lemon, lime, or a squeeze
of orange juice for a kick of flavor.

¾ cup olive oil

¼ cup balsamic vinegar

2 teaspoons dried oregano

Salt and black pepper to taste

In a bowl or small mason jar, whisk together the oil, vinegar, and oregano.
Season with salt and pepper. Store in the refrigerator. Shake or whisk
before using. You can play with the ratio of oil to vinegar to feed your
taste buds.

Per serving: 82 calories, 0 g protein, 0 g carbohydrates, 10 g total fat,
1.5 g saturated fat, 0 g fiber, 0 mg sodium

ANATOMY OF A HEALTHY SALAD

A salad bowl is like a blank canvas: Add the right stuff and you'll have a mouthwatering masterpiece. Here's intel for the tastiest, healthiest work of art.

Pick Pomegranate

Pomegranate seeds are naturally low in calories and high in antioxidants. Plus they add color!

Go Nuts

Fiber, fat, and protein give your salad more staying power.

Don't Fear Cheese

It's women's best source of calcium.

Add Eggs

The yolks' fat helps you absorb up to nine times more carotenoid antioxidants.

Mix Red and Green

A blend of lettuces may protect best against free radicals.

DIY Dressing

Mixing olive oil and vinegar is the easiest way to avoid extra sugar and chemical emulsifiers.

Sources: *Journal of Agricultural and Food Chemistry*; USDA National Nutrient Database for Standard Reference; *FASEB Journal*; *American Journal of Clinical Nutrition*; *Nature*

BREAKFAST

Easy Eggs Antigua

Makes 1 serving

Switch out your scrambled eggs for poached eggs seasoned with a hint of vinegar and your taste buds will rejoice!

1 teaspoon olive oil

1 whole wheat English muffin, toasted

½ cup frozen spinach

2 eggs

2 teaspoons white wine vinegar

Salt and black pepper to taste

1. Drizzle the olive oil over each open half of the toasted English muffin.

2. In a small, microwaveable bowl, microwave the spinach on high for 60 to 90 seconds, or until warm and wilted. Arrange the spinach on the toasted muffin halves.

3. Crack each egg into a separate small bowl or ramekin.

4. Fill a saucepan with a few inches of water, add the vinegar, and heat on high until the water starts to boil. Using the handle of a slotted spatula, stir the water in one direction until it's spinning around. While it's still spinning, carefully drop the eggs into the center of the whirlpool. Now turn off the heat and cover the pan. Allow the eggs to poach for 4 minutes.

5. Gently remove the eggs with a slotted spoon. Serve the eggs over the English muffin. Season with salt and pepper.

Per serving: 319 calories, 18 g protein, 27 g carbohydrates, 14 g total fat, 3 g saturated fat, 5 g fiber, 454 mg sodium

Apple-Cinnamon Quinoa Breakfast Bowl

Makes 2 servings

Quinoa is a total game changer in the morning—warm and filling, it's the perfect combination of protein and fiber to give your boring breakfast a boost!

½ cup uncooked quinoa (yields 1½ cups cooked)

1 cup water

½ small apple, diced, skin on (for fiber)

2 tablespoons golden raisins

¼ cup finely chopped walnuts

½ teaspoon ground cinnamon

1. Place the quinoa in a fine-mesh strainer and rinse it with cold running water. This will help remove any bitter flavors.

2. In a small pot, bring the quinoa and water to a boil. Reduce to the lowest heat setting, cover, and simmer for 15 to 20 minutes. Remove the pot from the heat and allow the quinoa to stand for 5 minutes, covered.

3. Stir in the apple, raisins, walnuts, and cinnamon. Serve warm. Stow leftovers in the fridge and reheat later—cooked quinoa keeps for up to 7 days.

Per serving: 349 calories, 10 g protein, 42 g carbohydrates, 12 g total fat, 0.5 g saturated fat, 6 g fiber, 8 mg sodium

Quinoa IQ

1. Quinoa is ready to serve when all the water is absorbed and the quinoa appears to have popped open, revealing a tiny dark center.

2. Red quinoa is best for cold salads, as it retains its shape better than white and black varieties.

3. Quinoa is considered a quick-cooking grain, so it's ideal for a time-crunch meal.

4. Rinse quinoa before cooking to remove a bitter plant residue of saponins known to keep insects away.

5. Quinoa contains all nine essential amino acids and is considered a complete protein.

Greek Yogurt and Oats

Makes 1 serving

This simple but filling breakfast is ideal for a busy morning. When cooking seems like an exhausting test of your morning abilities, grab your oats and yogurt to go! Feel free to add pomegranate seeds or fresh or frozen berries for a sweet sensation.

1 packet plain instant oatmeal   ¾ cup plain, full-fat Greek yogurt

Prepare the oatmeal according to package directions. Allow the oatmeal to cool and mix in the yogurt.

Per serving: 259 calories, 24 g protein, 27 g carbohydrates, 6 g total fat, 3 g saturated fat, 3 g fiber, 135 mg sodium

OVER THE MOON WITH OATS

Oats can be a gluten-free grain. Just look for oatmeal labeled "gluten-free."

Avoid highly processed oats and look for instant oatmeal brands such as McCann's Irish Oatmeal or Better Oats.

When on the run, grab oatmeal from Starbucks, Pret A Manger, or even Jamba Juice.

LUNCH

Granny Smith Goat Cheese Sandwich

Makes 1 serving

Think of this as a "grown-up" grilled cheese. Grab two slices of whole wheat or sprouted-grain bread and indulge your inner child with this healthy upgrade to a classic.

2 slices sprouted-grain or whole wheat bread, toasted

2 ounces goat cheese

½ green apple, thinly sliced

1 ounce (about 24) almonds

Spread both slices of the toasted bread with goat cheese and place the apple slices on one side. Close the sandwich. Serve with a side of almonds for a dose of heart-healthy monounsaturated fats.

Per serving: 512 calories, 20 g protein, 57 g carbohydrates, 26 g total fat, 1 g saturated fat, 10 g fiber, 392 mg sodium

Your Midafternoon Munch

Nuts and fiber-rich foods like carrots are filling, so you'll feel satisfied and less tempted to raid the vending machine.

Roasted Veggies with Chicken Sausage

Makes 2 servings

Your kitchen is your laboratory. Have fun and experiment with what vegetables are in season—there's no right or wrong in the kitchen! Switching out your fresh vegetables adds versatility to this dish and refreshes the taste each time you make it.

3 cloves garlic, pressed

1 medium sweet potato, chopped

8 small cipollini onions, halved

½ pound Brussels sprouts, trimmed and halved

3 tablespoons olive oil, or as needed

2 teaspoons dried oregano

Dash of ground red pepper, garlic powder, onion powder, black pepper, or herbes de Provence (optional)

1 green bell pepper, chopped

2 precooked chicken sausages, each sliced into 6–8 pieces

1. Preheat the oven to 400°F.

2. In a roasting pan, mix the garlic, sweet potato, onions, and Brussels sprouts. Drizzle with the olive oil and oregano. Add the ground red pepper, garlic powder, onion powder, black pepper, or herbes de Provence (if using) or adjust the seasonings according to your preference. Mix the ingredients well with a wooden spoon, coating with herbs and oil.

3. Transfer the vegetables to the oven and roast for 30 minutes, mixing occasionally.

4. Add the bell pepper and sausages and roast for another 15 minutes.

    VARIATION: *Try substituting tofu for the chicken sausage for an alternative, vegetarian source of protein.*

    Per serving: 425 calories, 21 g protein, 47 g carbohydrates, 24 g total fat, 5 g saturated fat, 9 g fiber, 382 mg sodium

Game Changer

For the Grill

Brooklyn Cured Chicken Garlic Sausage

Bilinski's Italian Herb Chicken Sausage

Tuna-Filled Pita
with a Side of Oreos

Makes 1 serving

This is your opportunity to learn how to eat all foods in balance with your body's needs. Give yourself permission and patience while learning how to eat mindfully.

1 can (5 ounces) chunk light tuna in water, no salt added

1–2 tablespoons country-style Dijon mustard

2 tablespoons finely chopped celery

¼ cup diced fresh pineapple or 2 tablespoons dried cranberries (optional)

Black pepper to taste

1 whole wheat pita

2 or 3 Oreo-like cookies such as Chips Ahoy!, Back to Nature, or Newman's Own

1. In a medium bowl, mix together the tuna, mustard, celery, and pine-apple or cranberries (if using). Season with pepper.

2. Fill the pita with tuna and choose your side of cookies. Be sure to refer to Chapter 8, "Skill Builder: How to Eat an Oreo."

Per serving: 519 calories, 28 g protein, 47 g carbohydrates, 7 g total fat, 1.5 g saturated fat, 7 g fiber, 990 mg sodium

Don't Mess with Mercury

When choosing your can of tuna, be sure to minimize your mercury exposure by choosing light tuna rather than albacore.

DINNER

PHASE 2: Time Crunch

Orecchiette with Pesto and Sausage

Makes 2 servings

Orecchiette is an easy way to upgrade a boring old plate of pasta to pure deliciousness. Mix with a fresh pesto sauce and enjoy!

1 cup uncooked whole wheat orecchiette pasta (yields about 1½ cups cooked)

2 cloves garlic, minced

2 Italian chicken sausages, each sliced into 6–8 pieces

¼ cup Le Grand Garden pesto or your favorite pesto

Black pepper to taste

1. Bring 2 quarts of water to a boil and add the pasta. Cook the pasta for about 11 minutes, or until al dente. Rinse the pasta under cool water while draining in a colander. Transfer to a bowl and set aside.

2. Lightly spray olive oil in a large skillet over medium heat. Add the garlic and cook, stirring frequently, for 1 minute. Add the sausages, cooking for 4 to 5 minutes, or until brown. Mix in the pasta and pesto and cook for 2 more minutes. Season with pepper.

Per serving: 405 calories, 20 g protein, 46 g carbohydrates, 16 g total fat, 1.5 g saturated fat, 6 g fiber, 541 mg sodium

Game Changer

Pesto

When buying pesto rather than making it, choose Le Grand Garden pesto. It's also vegan-friendly!

BBQ Chicken with Sweet Potato and Roasted Broccoli

Makes 2 servings

This is an easy meal to model when eating out. Think: carbohydrate, protein, and fat. The potato and broccoli are your carb sources, chicken is your protein, and olive oil is a source of healthy fats.

Barbecue Sauce

⅓ cup ketchup (check the label to ensure high-fructose corn syrup is not an ingredient)

1 tablespoon water

1 tablespoon cider vinegar

2 teaspoons Worcestershire sauce

2 tablespoons light brown sugar

¼ teaspoon onion powder

¼ teaspoon black pepper

2 chicken breasts (5 ounces each)

½ cup Barbecue Sauce

2 cups broccoli florets, brushed with olive oil

Sea salt to taste

1 medium sweet potato

Avoid an Energy Zapper

Too many calories can leave you lethargic; too few and you're flagging without the fuel and nutrients you need. Aim for 500 calories at lunch and 200 for snacks. At lunch, mix carbs and protein with healthy fats like those in olive oil.

1. Preheat the oven to 425°F. Line two 9" x 13" baking sheets with foil.

2. **To make the sauce:** In a small bowl, whisk together the ketchup, water, vinegar, Worcestershire sauce, sugar, onion powder, and black pepper.

3. Place the chicken on one of the baking sheets and brush with barbecue sauce. Roast for 40 minutes on the lower rack of the oven, brushing with sauce again at the halfway point. Place the brushed broccoli on the second baking sheet, sprinkle with sea salt, and roast for 3 to 5 minutes on the upper rack, or until crunchy.

4. Meanwhile, clean the sweet potato and poke holes in it with a fork. Microwave it for 5 minutes on high and let it cool. Cut it in half and let it roast with the broccoli for 2 to 3 minutes to get a little crunchy.

Per serving: 338 calories, 35 g protein, 36 g carbohydrates, 5 g total fat, 2 g saturated fat, 4 g fiber, 600 mg sodium

Don't Kill the Broccoli

Cook the tiny "trees" for just 3 to 5 minutes. Overcooking can decrease broccoli's star compounds, including glucosinolates, which have been linked to cancer protection. Steam it, rather than stir-frying or boiling, which deplete its benefits whatever the cooking time.

Garlicky Shrimp with Spaghetti Squash and Spinach

Makes 2 servings

Just looking at this dish will decrease your cortisol! The beautiful, bright mix of yellow squash, luscious greens, and pink shrimp makes all five of your senses do the happy dance.

1 small spaghetti squash (3 pounds)

1 tablespoon olive oil

½ pound deveined, uncooked shrimp with tails removed

3 cloves garlic, minced

1 package (10 ounces) fresh baby spinach

½ cup halved plum cherry tomatoes

¼ cup shredded Romano cheese

Go Light, Sleep Tight

A calorie-light, nutritious dinner makes it easier to sleep more deeply and wake up ready to go. That's probably because heavy meals appear to disrupt REM sleep (the most restful kind) and take longer to digest, so the body stays slightly revved as it tries to deal with that rich chicken potpie.

1. Cut the spaghetti squash in half width-wise. Scoop out the seeds and discard.

2. Steam each half of the squash. Place the squash in a microwaveable dish cut side down in 1″ of water. Microwave on high for about 7 minutes. Let cool cut side up for about 5 minutes. It should be slightly al dente.

3. Using a fork, scrape out the flesh so it looks like spaghetti. Transfer the strands into a clean bowl and set aside.

4. Heat the olive oil in a large sauté pan over medium heat. Add the shrimp and flip when the bottom side becomes opaque, 2 to 3 minutes. Add the minced garlic to the shrimp, stir for 1 minute, and then add the spinach. Mix until all ingredients are combined. Once the spinach is wilted, add the tomatoes to the mixture and let cook for 1 minute. Mix in the spaghetti squash and let all the veggies' juices blend together.

5. Divide the mixture evenly into 2 bowls and serve sprinkled with cheese.

Per serving: 461 calories, 34 g protein, 56 g carbohydrates, 15 g total fat, 3 g saturated fat, 4 g fiber, 456 mg sodium

Tiny but Mighty

Shrimp boast 7 grams of lean protein per ounce (look for wild, domestic caught) plus selenium, a mineral that's essential to a humming metabolism.

BREAKFAST

Simple Mediterranean Breakfast

Makes 1 serving

This dish is a combination of authentic Mediterranean ingredients that bring a bold, unique flavor to your morning meal. Dig in and imagine you're dining in a café along the coast; this dish will fuel that creativity and give you the nutrients you need to keep it humming all day.

1 teaspoon olive oil

2 eggs

1 serving Israeli Salad

1 ounce feta cheese

1.   Warm the olive oil in a skillet over medium heat.

2.   Crack and add the eggs and stir for 2 to 3 minutes, or until cooked. Serve immediately with a side of Israeli Salad topped with feta cheese.

Per serving: 346 calories, 18 g protein, 8 g carbohydrates, 26 g total fat, 8 g saturated fat, 2 g fiber, 459 mg sodium

Nutrition facts include Israeli Salad.

Say Cheese!

One ounce of feta has about 10 percent of the fat-burning calcium you need in a day.

Israeli Salad

Makes 2 servings

Wake up your taste buds with a tart, juicy salad that pairs well with savory breakfast foods for a well-balanced (and filling) meal.

2 medium English cucumbers, skin on and chopped

1 medium Roma tomato, chopped

¼ cup diced red onion

¼ cup chopped parsley

1 tablespoon olive oil

Salt and black pepper to taste

In a medium bowl, combine the cucumbers, tomato, onion, parsley, and olive oil. Divide the mixture in half and save one portion for another morning this week. Season with salt and pepper.

Per serving: 166 calories, 2 g protein, 10 g carbohydrates, 14 g total fat, 2 g saturated fat, 2 g fiber, 17 mg sodium

SIDESTEP THE SUGAR SPIKERS

Remember your mantra: All foods are A-okay, but keep in mind that starches and sweets tend to spike your blood sugar and insulin response, slowing down your fast track to a leaner, healthier body. Here are some common culprits to be sure to mix with proteins and fats while decreasing the overall portions.

Bananas	Doughnuts	White rice
Biscuits	Grapes	Soda
Candy	Ice cream	Sweet tea
Chips	Juices	White bread
Cookies	Pasta	

Vanilla Chia Pudding with Berries

Makes 1 serving

This recipe is inspired by Laura Iu, RDN and creator of dowhatiulove.com. Chia is a great source of fat and protein. Pair it with vanilla and berries to satisfy your sweet tooth!

¾ cup unsweetened almond milk

½ teaspoon pure vanilla extract

1 tablespoon honey, raw and local

¼ cup chia seeds

½ cup fresh berries, whole or mashed

1. In a small bowl or jar, combine the milk, vanilla extract, and honey.

2. Using a fork, whisk in the chia seeds. Let the mixture stand for 5 minutes and then stir to distribute any seeds that have settled.

3. Cover and refrigerate for at least 1 hour, or until the mixture develops a puddinglike consistency. Mix before serving.

4. To serve, top with berries for natural sweetness in every bite. Know that you can always adjust the consistency of the pudding: more milk for a thinner consistency and less milk for thicker. You can make this pudding ahead of time and store it in the refrigerator for up to 2 or 3 days.

Per serving: 387 calories, 19 g protein, 42 g carbohydrates, 20 g total fat, 0 g saturated fat, 20 g fiber, 146 mg sodium

Protein-Packed Toast

Makes 1 serving

Love cream cheese and lox? Try this instead: The added eggs, hummus, and cucumbers create the perfect balance of protein on your morning toast.

2 tablespoons hummus

2 slices sprouted-grain or whole wheat bread, toasted

¼ cup sliced cucumber

2 hard-cooked eggs, sliced

Spread the hummus on the toasted bread. Top with the cucumber and eggs.

Per serving: 315 calories, 21 g protein, 28 g carbohydrates, 13 g total fat, 3.5 g saturated fat, 6 g fiber, 494 mg sodium

LUNCH

Make Me Greek Salad Wrap

Makes 1 serving

Enjoy this wrap as an all-veggie option or top with your favorite protein source—grilled chicken, shrimp, or tofu.

- 1 cup chopped leafy greens of your choice (kale or baby spinach)
- ¼ cup chopped red bell pepper
- ¼ cup diced cucumber
- ½ small Roma tomato, chopped
- 2 tablespoons crumbled feta cheese

- ¼ cup pitted black olives
- 1 tablespoon Body Clock Vinaigrette (page 145)
- 1 whole wheat tortilla
- 4 ounces grilled chicken, shrimp, or tofu (optional)

In a medium bowl, toss the leafy greens, bell pepper, cucumber, tomato, cheese, olives, and Body Clock Vinaigrette. Spoon the vegetable mixture onto the tortilla, layer with a protein of choice (if desired), and roll up.

Per serving with 4 ounces of chicken: 495 calories, 38 g protein, 26 g carbohydrates, 27 g total fat, 6 g saturated fat, 5 g fiber, 586 mg sodium

Veggie Burger with a Side of Fruit and "Sometimes Food"

Makes 1 serving

We're not all perfect—but that's no reason to abandon your diet for imperfect food! Before you rush out the door, whip together this easy-to-assemble lunch for a quick, indulgent option that keeps you from falling completely off track.

1 veggie burger

Greens, tomatoes, sprouts, avocado, onions, cheese (optional toppings)

1 whole wheat bun or English muffin

1 fruit of your choice

2 Oreo-like cookies (or any "sometimes food" of your choice, such as a serving of chips or a small granola bar)

Prepare the veggie burger according to package directions. Serve with your favorite toppings on a bun or English muffin. Enjoy your fruit and "sometimes food" as sides. Eat mindfully and feel good knowing you're mastering the art of eating all foods!

*Per serving: 400 calories, 12 g protein, 65 g carbohydrates, 12 g total fat, 3 g saturated fat, 9 g fiber, 747 mg sodium

Nutrition facts include ½ cup strawberries and 2 Oreos. Toppings are not included.

Game Changers

No-Meat Sliders

Dr. Praeger's California Veggie Burger

Amy's Quarter Pound Veggie Burger

Hilary's Gluten Free World's Best Veggie Burger

Tomato-Basil-Mozzarella Sandwich with Tomato Soup

Makes 1 serving

Whether you're stuck without lunch or you want to re-create the same delicious meal you can find at Panera, here's a recipe for decadent flatbread to go.

1 cup canned tomato soup (we love Amy's Light in Sodium Cream of Tomato soup)

2 slices bread, toasted

1 tablespoon Body Clock Vinaigrette (page 145)

½ small Roma tomato, thinly sliced

3 large fresh basil leaves

1 ounce sliced mozzarella cheese

Black pepper to taste

1. Prepare the soup according to package directions.

2. Meanwhile, place the toasted bread on a flat surface and drizzle each slice with Body Clock Vinaigrette. Top evenly with tomato, basil leaves, and mozzarella. Season with pepper. Close the sandwich and enjoy with a side of soup.

Per serving: 471 calories, 19 g protein, 54 g carbohydrates, 24 g total fat, 7 g saturated fat, 8 g fiber, 667 mg sodium

Avocado Size Matters

Forgive the buzzkill, embrace the truth. If you're adding avocado to your burger, consider this: One proper serving (2 tablespoons) is roughly the size of a dental floss container (50 calories, 5 g fat, 2 g fiber).

DINNER

Simply Satisfying Salmon with Garlicky Haricots Verts

Makes 2 servings

If you don't like fish, I dare you to try this recipe! The mustard and bread crumbs bring it to a whole new level. Be sure to sit down to this meal and truly take in the colors, the mouthfeel, and the nutrients. Think of the omega-3 fatty acids helping to conduct nerve signals and decrease the inflammation in your body.

2 wild salmon fillets (4 ounces each)

2 tablespoons mustard

1 tablespoon bread crumbs

2 teaspoons olive oil

2 cloves garlic, minced

½ pound haricots verts (frozen or fresh), tips removed

½ cup cooked whole wheat orzo

½ cup canned lentils, drained

1. Preheat the oven to 350°F. Line a 9" x 13" baking sheet with foil.

2. Place the salmon on the baking sheet and spread the mustard on the fillets. Next coat with a layer of bread crumbs. Cover with a foil tent and bake for 10 minutes.

3. Meanwhile, heat the oil in a large pan over medium heat. Add the garlic and cook, stirring frequently, for 2 minutes, or until fragrant. Add the haricots verts and cook, stirring frequently, for 8 minutes. Add the cooked pasta and lentils. Mix well.

4. Undo the foil tent from around the salmon and broil for 5 minutes, or until the salmon is flaky and pink (not red). Serve the salmon immediately with the haricots verts.

Per serving: 520 calories, 47 g protein, 60 g carbohydrates, 11 g total fat, 2 g saturated fat, 20 g fiber, 454 mg sodium

Fast Chicken Fajitas

Makes 2 servings

Bold flavors make these fajitas taste so good you can enjoy them with or without the tortillas. But what's even better is that they're super quick and easy to prepare!

2 tablespoons non-GMO canola oil

¼ cup thinly sliced onion

2 cloves garlic, pressed and minced

2 chicken breasts (4 ounces each), thinly sliced

½ cup frozen unsalted corn

1 cup frozen mixed bell peppers

2 whole grain tortillas

2 tablespoons sour cream (dairy or nondairy)

¼ cup salsa (bean or tomato)

1. Warm the oil in a large skillet over medium heat. Add the onion, stirring for 2 minutes, then add the garlic.

2. Add the chicken slices to the skillet. Once the chicken is slightly pink in the center, add the corn and peppers. Cook, stirring frequently, for 5 to 7 minutes, or until the veggies are cooked through.

3. Warm the tortillas in the microwave for about 20 seconds or in a pan over low heat.

4. Spread a tablespoon of sour cream down the center of each tortilla. Then spread 2 tablespoons of salsa over the sour cream. Spoon the chicken and pepper combo down the center of the tortilla. Roll, and serve while hot.

Per serving: 510 calories, 42 g protein, 32 g carbohydrates, 23 g total fat, 3 g saturated fat, 5 g fiber, 501 mg sodium

Pasta and Sautéed Brussels Sprouts with Pine Nuts and Parmesan

Makes 2 servings

Brussels sprouts are one of the trendiest and healthiest veggies to be found on restaurant menus across the states. They're super filling and therefore ideal to eat with a food like pasta that may be harder to portion manage.

1 cup uncooked whole wheat orecchiette pasta (yields about 1½ cups cooked)

3 tablespoons olive oil, divided

2 cloves garlic, pressed

½ pound Brussels sprouts, trimmed and halved

4 tablespoons pine nuts

Salt and black pepper to taste

¼ cup grated Parmesan cheese

1.   Bring 2 quarts of water to a rolling boil. Add the pasta to the water and stir. Cook for about 11 minutes, or until al dente. Rinse the pasta under cool water while draining in a colander. Transfer to a bowl and set aside.

2.   While the pasta is cooking, heat 2 tablespoons of the olive oil in a large skillet over medium heat. Add the garlic and cook, stirring frequently, for 2 minutes.

3.   Arrange the Brussels sprouts in the skillet, cut side down in a single layer. Cook the sprouts without turning them for 7 minutes and then add the pine nuts. Flip the sprouts and cook the underside, stirring, for about 5 minutes. Once the sprouts are crisp, tender, and golden brown, add the pasta.

4.   Drizzle the remaining tablespoon of olive oil onto the pasta and stir for 1 minute. Season with salt and pepper. Sprinkle each serving with about 2 tablespoons of grated Parmesan cheese and serve immediately.

Per serving: 540 calories, 14 g protein, 44 g carbohydrates, 34 g total fat, 5 g saturated fat, 8 g fiber, 195 mg sodium

DESSERT

PHASE 3: Make Me

'Nana Chocolate Peanut Butter Ice Cream*

Makes 1 serving

Pop a banana, sans the peel, into your freezer the night before and build this delicious dessert!

1 medium ripe banana

2 tablespoons natural nut butter, no added salt, stored at room temperature

1 tablespoon mini dark chocolate chips

1 tablespoon chopped unsalted almonds

1. Peel the banana and stick it in the freezer for 3 hours or ideally overnight to freeze solid.

2. Chop the frozen banana into 1" to 2" pieces and toss into a food processor or Vitamix. Pulse the pieces continuously, until the banana has a crumbly texture. Use a spatula to scrape down the sides of the food processor and keep blending till your banana starts to look gooey, with a few chunks. Repeat the steps of blending and scraping the sides of the processor until the mixture resembles a creamy soft-serve ice cream texture.

3. Transfer your 'nana ice cream to a bowl, drizzle with nut butter, and sprinkle with chocolate chips and chopped almonds. You can either serve this immediately or, for the texture of traditional ice cream, place the bowl back in the freezer for about 15 minutes, or until the desired consistency is achieved.

Per serving: 384 calories, 10 g protein, 39 g carbohydrates, 21 g total fat, 4 g saturated fat, 6 g fiber, 1 mg sodium

This recipe is courtesy of dowhatiulove.com.

The Body Clock Diet Workouts

EXERCISES FOR PHASES 1, 2, AND 3 THAT RESPECT YOUR PRECIOUS TIME

Always do what you are afraid to do.
—RALPH WALDO EMERSON

When your body clock becomes discombobulated by, say, watching *House of Cards* back-to-back-to-back at 11:30 p.m. or crossing time zones in an airplane, exercise can help reset it.

Regular exercise not only strengthens muscles, it can strengthen your circadian rhythms by reducing stress, increasing daytime alertness, boosting the immune system, and bringing on sleepiness at night.

Studies by the National Sleep Foundation have shown that exercise improves the quantity *and* quality of sleep. Remember, enough sleep and good-quality sleep are hugely important because slumber time is when your body expends a lot of calories on recovery and repair and building lean, strong muscle. Sweat-induced, better sleep may be due to those feel-good endorphins that exercise is so famous for triggering. But new research in the journal *Medicine and Science in Sports and Exercise* found that there may be something stronger and longer lasting at work: The soothing effect may result from the self-confidence regular exercise provides.

That should make you even more motivated to get on a workout routine. Just like creating structure for meals, scheduling regular exercise can help keep the beat for your internal clock. The two keys are consistency and simplicity, says BJ Gaddour, fitness director of *Men's Health* magazine and author of *Your Body Is Your Barbell.* "All you need is your body, and maybe a pair of dumbbells, for an amazing workout at home," he says.

He's right. By planning a weekly schedule of body-weight workouts and fast-paced cardio intervals you can do anywhere, you'll never have to step inside a gym. "Journaling your workouts week after week shows progress, instills confidence, and makes exercise part of your lifestyle," Gaddour says. "You'll feel unstoppable."

And that's the secret to lasting weight loss.

TIMED WORKOUTS TO FIT ANY SCHEDULE

People often avoid exercise because they think it's impossible to fit into their busy schedules. But structure here can be your savior. By building a menu of exercise routines of varying lengths and intensities, you can slot them into your daily life no matter what your day throws at you.

You've heard the long-recommended advice to get 30 minutes of exercise a day? It's still valid, but ongoing research continues to prove that even less time can be more beneficial if you increase the intensity of the physical effort in short, frequent bursts. This is what's known as interval training, and it can be done using body-weight circuits, dumbbell strength routines, and workouts on cardio equipment like stationary cycles and ellipticals, and even by walking. The key is *short* and *vigorous.* Dozens of studies have found that these high-intensity interval training (or HIIT)

DOUBLE UP AGAINST DIABETES

Harvard University researchers found that combining resistance training with aerobic activity for a total of 300 minutes per week can reduce your risk of type 2 diabetes by up to 59 percent.

workouts lower blood pressure and control blood sugar better than even hour-long, slo-mo workouts. In fact, researchers in Denmark found that women who completed shorter intense workouts burned more calories than those who logged lengthier ones. Even cooler: You can stack workouts. In other words, if you want the health-boosting benefits of a full 30 minutes of exercise, you can do three 10-minute bouts or one 10-minute brisk interval walk in the morning and a 20-minute strength workout in the afternoon. The results come from the cumulative effort. It all adds up. And the sheer versatility of workout options means you can adapt exercise to your available time without upsetting the rhythm of your day.

On the following pages you'll find eight effective calorie-burning, muscle-toning, health-improving workouts of various types and lengths. We will start exercise with Phase 1 of the plan, but if you aren't ready for that and want to concentrate all your effort on mastering the three body clock resets, that's fine. Simply start the Phase 1 workout schedule on page 176 when you reach Phase 2.

Try to do three Body Clock Diet strength workouts per week and at least one high-intensity interval training workout. Also try to move your body more every day with walking, the Body Clock Energy Peanuts, and Yoga in a Flash practice in this chapter.

You can arrange your workout schedule however you like as long as you leave a day in between strength workouts. See the following pages for a sample.

Phase 1 Workout Schedule (2 weeks)

Every Morning

The Eye-Opener (page 179)

Do 1 set of 4 exercises for 3 minutes before breakfast.

Monday

Total-Body Tone-at-Home Circuit (page 184)

Marching Glute Bridge, 10 to 12 reps

Alternating Reverse Lunge, 10 to 12 reps

Plank Pushup, 10 to 12 reps

Skater Hop, 10 to 12 reps

Tuesday (OPTIONAL)

1-mile recovery walk

Wednesday

Better Butt and Thighs Mini-Band Moves (page 189)

SUPERSET 1 (2 SETS)

Mini-Band Glute Bridge, 8 to 12 reps

Mini-Band Lateral Shuffle, 10 reps in each direction

REST for 60 seconds

SUPERSET 2 (2 SETS)

Mini-Band Squat, 15 to 20 reps

Mini-Band Knee Raise, 10 to 12 reps

Thursday

Rest or light cardio (walking or biking) for 30 minutes

Friday

Total-Body Tone-at-Home Circuit

Saturday

HIIT Reset (high-intensity interval training) for 30 minutes (page 194)

Sunday

Off (Use Yoga in a Flash [page 219] any day.)

Phase 2 Workout Schedule (2 weeks)

Every Morning

The Eye-Opener

Do 1 set of 4 exercises for 3 minutes before breakfast.

Monday

Dumbbell Strength Circuit 1 (page 196)

Dumbbell Squat, 30 seconds

Pushup, 30 seconds

Dumbbell Bent-Over Row, 30 seconds plus piston finisher

Goblet Split Squat, 30 seconds with each leg

Dumbbell Pushup-Position Row, 30 seconds

Dumbbell Overhead Press, 30 seconds

Tuesday

Rest or light cardio activity such as walking or biking for 30 minutes

Wednesday

Dumbbell Strength Circuit 2 (page 203)

Goblet Squat, 8 to 12 reps

Hammer Curl to Press, 8 to 12 reps

Dumbbell Deadlift, 8 to 12 reps

Single-Arm Dumbbell Row and Twist, 10 reps with each arm

Dumbbell Pullover, 8 to 12 reps

Thursday

Better Butt and Thighs Mini-Band Moves

Friday

Dumbbell Strength Circuit 1

Saturday

HIIT Reset (high-intensity interval training) for 30 minutes

Sunday

Off (Use Yoga in a Flash [page 219] any day.)

Phase 3 Workout Schedule (2 weeks)

Every Morning

The Eye-Opener

Do 1 set before breakfast for 3 minutes.

Monday

The Fat-Burner Superset (45 minutes) (page 209)

Warm up with jumping jacks or rope jumping for 5 minutes.

SUPERSET 1 (2 SETS)	SUPERSET 3 (2 SETS)
Clean and Press, 8 to 10 reps	Yoga Pushup, 8 to 10 reps
Power Squat, 10 reps	Bench Press, 8 to 10 reps
REST for 2 minutes	REST for 2 minutes

SUPERSET 2 (2 SETS)	SUPERSET 4 (2 SETS)
Curtsy Lunge, 8 to 10 reps on each side	Jump Power Lunge, 20 jumps
Lateral Lunge, 8 to 10 reps on each side	Double Reverse Lunge, 10 reps on each side
REST for 2 minutes	REST for 2 minutes

Tuesday

Rest or light cardiovascular activity like walking or biking for 30 minutes

Wednesday

Total-Body Tone-at-Home Circuit

Thursday

On and Off (high-intensity interval training) for 20 minutes (page 218)

Friday

The Fat-Burner Superset

Saturday

Fun exercise such as hiking, biking, tennis, etc., for 1+ hours

Sunday

Off (Use Yoga in a Flash [page 219] any day.)

3 MINUTES

THE EYE-OPENER

A cardiovascular quickie first thing in the morning can speed up alertness and jump-start your metabolism for the day. The Eye-Opener is a total-body blaster that hits all the major muscle groups, and its fast-paced, up-and-down movements will crank your cardiovascular response in about 60 seconds. The Eye-Opener is made up of four exercises—the Walking Lunge, Squat, Prone Cobra, and Plank with Leg Lift—that are performed as two combination moves back-to-back. Catch your breath between the combos if you need to, but work up to doing this 3-minute drill with no rest. Because this microworkout is so brief, you can do it every day, even on your main strength-training days.

WALKING LUNGE

MUSCLES WORKED
Quadriceps, glutes (butt), calves, and lower back

STARTING POSITION

Stand with your feet hip width apart, hands on hips.

THE MOVE

Step your right foot forward and bend your knees to lower your body until your right thigh is nearly parallel to the ground. Pause a second, and as you stand, push off your back foot, step your left foot forward, and dip into a lunge. Continue moving forward, alternating legs for 10 reps. (If you don't have room in your home to do walking lunges, step back to the starting position after each lunge.)

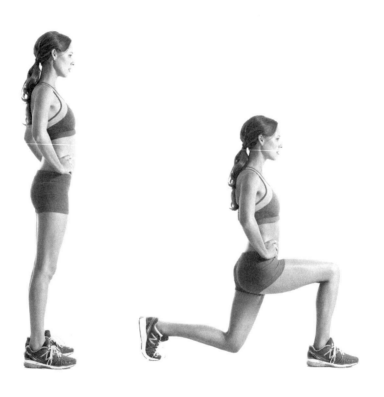

SQUAT

MUSCLES WORKED
Quadriceps, glutes, hamstrings, calves

STARTING POSITION

After the last walking lunge rep stand straight and step
your feet out so they're shoulder width apart for the body-weight squat. Raise your
hands behind your head with your fingers lightly touching your head or ears.

THE MOVE

Initiate the squat by sitting your butt back as if trying to close a door behind you with
your tush and bending your knees. Lower slowly until both thighs are parallel to the
floor or lower. Do as many reps as you can in 30 seconds.

Don't rest. Go right into the Prone Cobra (page 182).

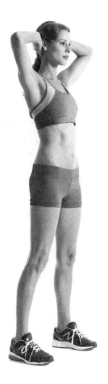
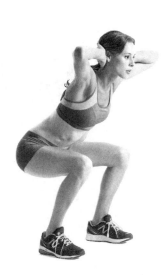

Energy Peanuts

Take the stairs anytime
you're traveling less than
four floors.

PRONE COBRA

MUSCLES WORKED

Lower back; core, including obliques; chest; and shoulders

STARTING POSITION

Lie facedown on the floor with your arms next to your sides, palms down, and your legs straight behind you, toes pointed.

THE MOVE

Contract your lower back and butt muscles and raise your head, chest, arms, and legs off the floor. Simultaneously, rotate your arms so that your thumbs point toward the ceiling. Hold this position for 15 seconds, then lower your limbs and head to the floor and repeat the move, holding for another 15 seconds before moving on to the next exercise.

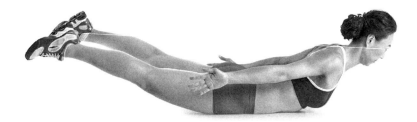

Energy Peanuts

Park in a spot farther away from your office to force yourself to walk a little more before and after work.

PLANK WITH LEG LIFT

STARTING POSITION

Get into a plank position, supporting your body between your elbows and forearms on the floor and the balls of your feet. Your elbows should be directly under your shoulders. Your back should be straight from your heels to your head. Tighten your core and make your body rigid by pulling your belly into your spine as if you were preparing to be punched in the tummy.

THE MOVE

Keeping your body rigid and legs straight, raise your left leg toward the ceiling until you feel the stretch in your lower back. Squeeze your left glute as hard as you can. Hold the top position for a second, then slowly release. Repeat with your right leg. That's one repetition. Alternate side to side for 10 reps. Try to avoid twisting your torso or allowing your belly to sag.

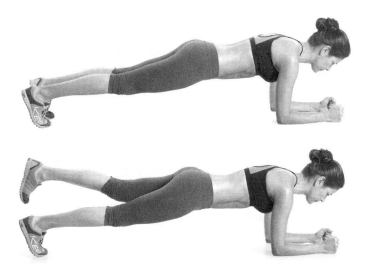

 Ticktock Tip

Three minutes can be all you need to increase your bloodflow and range of motion, improve mental performance, and reduce the risk for injury, says Andrea Fradkin, PhD, an associate professor of exercise science at Bloomsburg University in Pennsylvania.

15 MINUTES

TOTAL-BODY TONE-AT-HOME CIRCUIT

No equipment is required for this simple and quick routine, which makes it ideal for a home workout or one you can do in your hotel room when traveling. Do the following four exercises as a circuit. After completing an exercise, rest for 10 seconds and move on to the next. After completing all four moves, rest for 1 minute. Repeat the circuit two more times for a total of three.

MARCHING GLUTE BRIDGE

MUSCLES WORKED
Lower back, quadriceps, and core

STARTING POSITION

Lie faceup with your knees bent at 90-degree angles, feet on the floor and arms at your sides, palms down. Press through your heels to raise your hips and torso until your body forms a straight line from your knees to your shoulders. Brace your core.

THE MOVE

Keeping the knee bent, raise your right leg until your shin is parallel with the floor. Maintain a flexed ankle, toes pointing toward the ceiling. Hold for 3 seconds, then lower your foot to the floor and repeat with the left leg. That's 1 repetition. Do 10 to 12 reps.

FIT TIP

Don't raise your hips so high that you bow your lower back. That's hyperextension, and it can strain your muscles. But at the same time, don't allow your hips to sag toward the floor, which reduces the effectiveness of the exercise. If your core isn't strong enough to keep your hips up, take a rest and continue the reps when you've recovered.

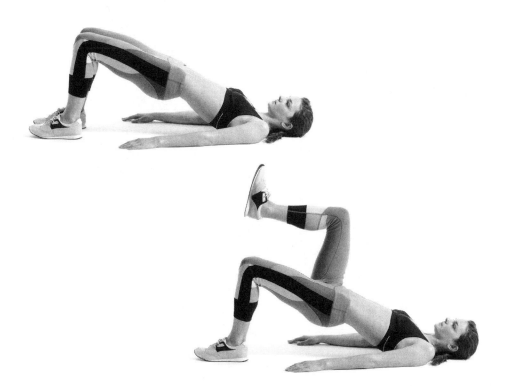

ALTERNATING REVERSE LUNGE

MUSCLES WORKED
Quadriceps, glutes, and hamstrings

STARTING POSITION

Stand with your feet hip width apart, hands clasped behind your head. Keep your chest up and eyes focused in front of you, not downward.

THE MOVE

Step back with your right leg and lower your body until your left knee is bent to 90 degrees. Pause a second, then push back up to the starting position. Repeat the exercise using your left leg. That's 1 repetition. Do 10 to 12 reps.

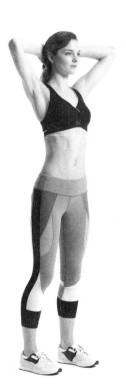

FIT TIP

In the lunge, your back knee should hover just about an inch over the floor. Be sure that your front knee does not extend farther than your toes.

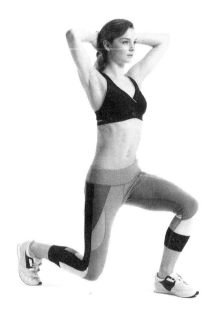

PLANK PUSHUP

MUSCLES WORKED
Core, chest, shoulders, and arms

STARTING POSITION

Get into a plank position with your forearms on the floor, elbows directly under your shoulders, and legs extended behind you. Look at the floor. Your body should form a line from your heels to your head. Brace your core.

THE MOVE

Raise your right arm and place your right hand flat on the floor and then your left hand, straightening your arms into pushup position. Return to the starting position by lowering onto your right, then left forearms. That's 1 repetition. On the next rep, lead with your left hand and continue alternating this way for 10 to 12 repetitions.

FIT TIP

Do this exercise on a rug or yoga mat to cushion your elbows and forearms.

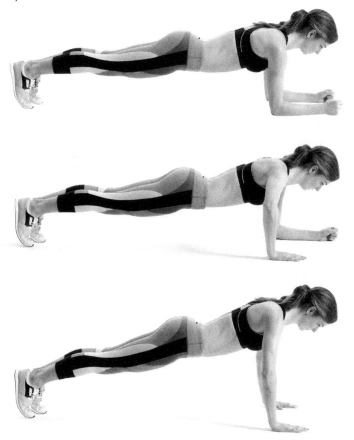

SKATER HOP

MUSCLES WORKED

Calves, hip flexors, and cardiovascular system

STARTING POSITION

Stand with feet hip width apart, knees and back slightly bent in an athletic stance. Give yourself some room to move laterally.

THE MOVE

This should be done aggressively. Cross your right leg behind your left and lower into a half-squat, your left arm out to the side, right arm across your hips. Immediately hop to the right and switch your legs and arms, swinging your right arm out and your left arm across your hips. That's 1 repetition. Continue hopping quickly, alternating from side to side for 10 to 12 total reps.

FIT TIP

As you master the move, concentrate on really pushing off the floor aggressively to hop as far as you can to the side while maintaining control and good form.

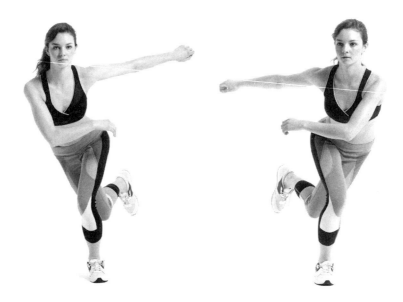

Energy Peanuts

Boost your confidence with index cards. Use them to write down brief short-term goals. Once you complete a goal, add the card to a stack. Having a pile of "done that" goals will spur future motivation.

15 MINUTES

BETTER BUTT AND THIGHS MINI-BAND MOVES

All you need for this workout is an inexpensive mini resistance band. (Until you buy one, you can do these moves without the band.) Do these four band moves as two supersets. In other words, perform all the reps of the first move, then immediately do the second move. That's one superset. Rest for up to 60 seconds following the second move. Repeat for a total of two supersets. Next, perform the third and fourth exercises as a superset in the same way.

MINI-BAND GLUTE BRIDGE

STARTING POSITION

Step into a mini band with both feet and position the band above your knees. Lie faceup on the floor, knees bent and the sides of your feet turned toward each other. Place your arms flat on the floor slightly angled away from your body.

THE MOVE

Raise your hips so your body forms a straight line from your knees to your shoulders, then drive your knees outward. Hold this position for 2 or 3 seconds, then bring your knees together and lower your butt to the floor. That's 1 rep. Do 8 to 12.

FIT TIP

To make this move harder, straighten one leg (foot elevated) and keep it parallel with the opposite thigh as you lift your hips. Do 4 to 6 reps with each leg.

Energy Peanuts

While standing in the checkout line at the grocery store, squeeze your buns. Not the bread, silly. Your butt, your glutes. Tense them for 5 seconds, then release and repeat. No one will ever know unless you're wearing yoga pants, which you shouldn't, please. Not while food shopping!

MINI-BAND LATERAL SHUFFLE

MUSCLES WORKED
Glutes, hips, thighs, abductors, and core

STARTING POSITION

Step into a mini band with both feet and position the band above your ankles. Step out against the band's resistance until your feet are about shoulder width apart. Bend your knees slightly into an athletic stance.

THE MOVE

Step your left foot out to the left followed by your right foot to the left, keeping your feet pointed forward. That's 1 repetition. Do 10 reps (lateral steps left). Then switch directions and repeat for 10 lateral steps to the right.

FIT TIP

Move slowly and in control. Hold your arms out in front of you with your elbows bent to keep your balance.

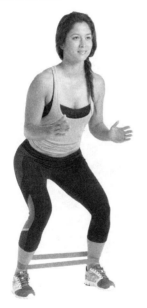
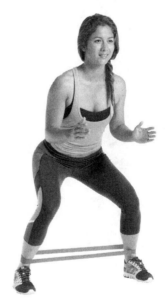

MINI-BAND SQUAT

<table>
<tr><td>MUSCLES WORKED</td></tr>
<tr><td>Glutes, quadriceps, and abductors</td></tr>
</table>

STARTING POSITION

Step into a mini band with both feet and position the band just above your knees. Stand straight with feet shoulder width apart.

THE MOVE

Push your hips back and bend your knees to lower your body as far as you can, spreading your knees outward against the band's resistance. Pause, then slowly push back to the starting position. That's 1 rep. Do 15 to 20.

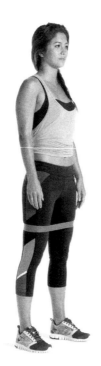
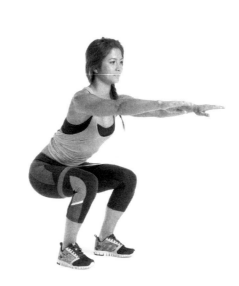

 Ticktock Tip

Popping new exercises into your workout can speed your heart rate from 60 to 80 percent of your max, so you burn an extra 120 calories an hour. Swap rowing in for running, free weights in for machines.

MINI-BAND KNEE RAISE

MUSCLES WORKED
Quadriceps and hip extensors

STARTING POSITION

Position a mini band around the toes of your athletic shoes and under their soles. Stand with your feet hip width apart, hands on your hips.

THE MOVE

Lift your left foot off the ground to bring your knee up to hip level, keeping the band around your shoe and your foot parallel to the floor. Pause a second, then return to the starting position and repeat, this time raising your right leg. That's 1 repetition. Do 10 to 12.

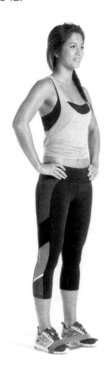 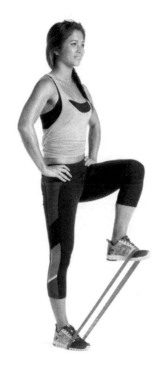

30 MINUTES

HIIT RESET

This interval cardio workout will boost your metabolic rate and leave your whole body feeling energized. Try to do this workout outside in the sunshine on a sidewalk, track, or bicycle. You can also do it inside on a treadmill or stationary bike. It's time based, so it'll help to wear a sports watch. The interval is broken into three effort levels: easy, hard, and moderate. Follow that pattern, one after another, without stopping to rest. After finishing the moderate segment, start over again with the easy segment until you've done each part three times. As your cardiovascular conditioning improves by Phases 2 and 3 of the Body Clock Diet program, try increasing the last segment (moderate) of round three to 8 minutes as a finisher.

EASY: 5 minutes—Go at an exercise intensity of 65 percent of your all-out effort.

HARD: 2 minutes—Go at an exercise intensity of about 85 percent of your all-out best effort.

MODERATE: 3 minutes—Go at an exercise intensity of about 75 percent of your best effort.

Ticktock Tip

Shave Minutes Off Your Gym Time

If you work out at home . . .

- Keep your weights out of the closet. If they're remotely in sight, you'll be more likely to use them.

- Stash your sneakers by the door to avoid searching prerun.

- Set your alarm to go off 10 minutes earlier. Morning workouts = just one shower a day.

If you work out at a gym . . .

- Avoid peak hours (even if it's just by 15 minutes).

- Leave your phone in your locker. Checking work e-mail or replying to a friend's text is bound to slow down your workout.

- Perfect the leggings look. Wear a tunic and leggings while running errands, then just change your top at the gym.

15 MINUTES

DUMBBELL STRENGTH CIRCUIT 1

This fast-paced circuit alternates lower- and upper-body muscle groups to burn more calories in less time. You'll need a sports watch or clock with a second hand for this one. Do the following exercises in order, completing as many repetitions of each exercise as you can in 30 seconds. After 30 seconds, go immediately into the next exercise without resting. Once you complete the sixth exercise, the overhead press, rest for 1 to 2 minutes, then repeat the circuit. Do a total of three circuits. You'll need a pair of dumbbells for most of these exercises. Use a weight that feels challenging; try starting with 8- to 12-pounders.

DUMBBELL SQUAT

MUSCLES WORKED
Quadriceps and calves

STARTING POSITION

Stand with your feet shoulder width apart and hold a pair of dumbbells at your sides, palms facing you.

THE MOVE

Sit your hips back and bend your knees to lower your body as far as you can, keeping your back flat and core tight. Press through your heels to return to the starting position. That's 1 rep. Do as many as possible in 30 seconds.

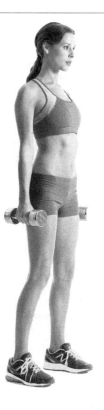

FIT TIP

Your upper body should stay as upright as possible.

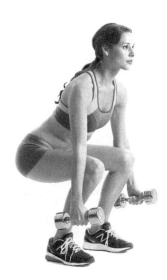

Energy Peanuts

Instead of e-mailing or texting, walk over to your coworker when you need to discuss something.

PUSHUP

MUSCLES WORKED

Chest and back

STARTING POSITION

Place your hands on the floor just outside your shoulders
and extend your legs behind you, body forming a straight line from head to heels.
Brace your core as if expecting a punch in the tummy.

THE MOVE

Keeping your back flat, lower your body toward the floor. Straighten your arms to
return to the starting position. That's 1 rep. Do as many as possible in 30 seconds.

FIT TIP

There are dozens and dozens of variations to the pushup. Experiment by moving your
hands closer together, farther apart, and even staggered. When pushups become
easy, try elevating your feet on a bench to increase the load on your chest.

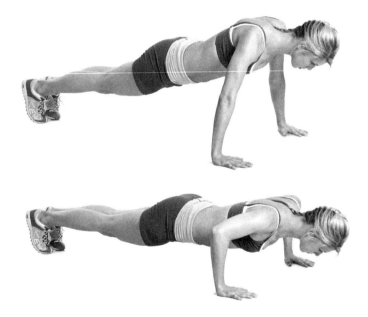

DUMBBELL BENT-OVER ROW

MUSCLES WORKED
Upper back

STARTING POSITION

Grab a pair of dumbbells and stand with your feet shoulder width apart, knees slightly bent. Bend forward from the hips until your chest is almost parallel to the floor, arms straight and weights in line with your shoulders.

THE MOVE

Pull the dumbbells up, squeezing your shoulder blades together. Pause, then return to the starting position. That's 1 repetition. Do as many as possible in 30 seconds.

FIT TIP

Add an extra challenge to this move. After completing 30 seconds of this exercise, take 10 more to do alternating dumbbell rows. Raise one dumbbell at a time, lowering it as you raise the other. Alternate quickly like pistons on an engine for 10 seconds.

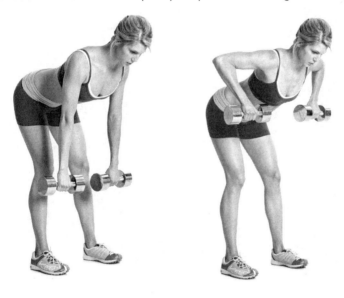

GOBLET SPLIT SQUAT

MUSCLES WORKED
Quadriceps and calves

STARTING POSITION

Stand with your feet together, then move your left foot
3 feet in front of your right, holding a dumbbell vertically
in front of your chest, hands clasping one end of the weight.

THE MOVE

Bend your knees to lower your body until your left thigh is parallel and your shin is perpendicular to the floor. Straighten your legs to return to the starting position. That's
1 rep. Continue for 30 seconds, then switch sides so your right foot is forward and
repeat for 30 seconds.

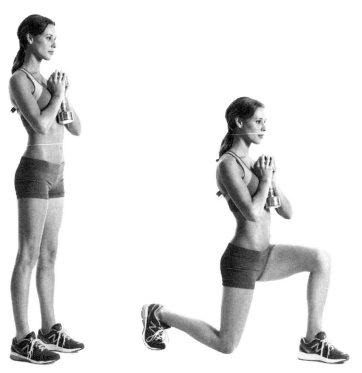

Energy Peanuts

For every 45 minutes you spend at your
desk or watching TV, spend 15 on your
feet. The US Endocrine Research Unit
found obese people sat for 164 minutes
longer per day than lean people.

DUMBBELL PUSHUP-POSITION ROW

MUSCLES WORKED
Chest, middle and upper back

STARTING POSITION

Get into a pushup position with your hands resting on the handles of two hexagonal dumbbells. (Use hex dumbbells, unlike the model shown below, so they won't roll under your weight.) The dumbbells should be directly under your shoulders. Spread your feet slightly more than hip width apart.

THE MOVE

Brace your abs as you pull one dumbbell toward your waist. Pause, lower the weight, then repeat with the other arm. That's 1 rep. As you continue, make sure your hips don't sag. Do as many as you can in 30 seconds.

FIT TIP

If you find your torso twisting as you do this exercise, spread your feet slightly wider for better balance.

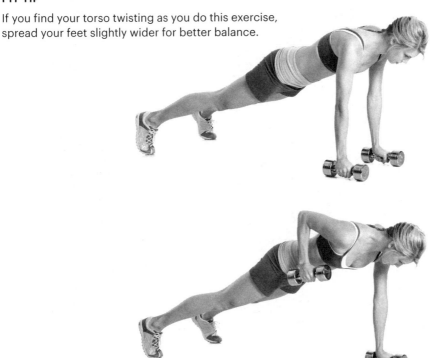

DUMBBELL OVERHEAD PRESS

STARTING POSITION

Hold a pair of dumbbells just outside your shoulders, palms facing each other. Brace your core.

THE MOVE

Press the weights directly overhead until your arms are completely straight. Lock out your elbows. Pause, then slowly lower back to the starting position. That's 1 rep. Do as many as you can in 30 seconds.

FIT TIP

Holding dumbbells with palms facing each other is called a neutral grip. This grip often reduces stress on the wrists.

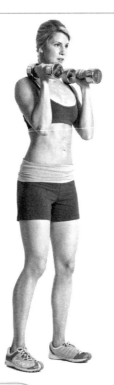
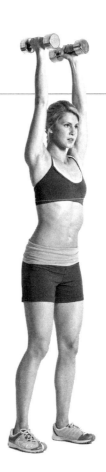

Energy Peanuts

Work out with your guy; couples who train together are 34 percent more likely to stick to their workouts.

20 MINUTES

DUMBBELL STRENGTH CIRCUIT 2

This speedy circuit will spike your metabolism and keep it elevated for hours afterward. If you must rest, go ahead, but the key to this workout is pushing yourself hard, so try to complete it with little to no rest between exercises. Do all reps of one exercise, then move directly to the next. After the fifth exercise, repeat the entire circuit for a total of four circuits. Make it your goal to complete the workout in 20 minutes. For this one you'll need a sports watch or clock with a second hand, a pair of dumbbells, and an exercise bench.

GOBLET SQUAT

MUSCLES WORKED
Quads and glutes

STARTING POSITION

Stand with your feet hip width apart and hold a dumbbell
vertically in front of your chest, hands clasping one end of the weight, elbows pointing
toward the floor.

THE MOVE

Push your hips back and bend your knees to lower into a squat. Your elbows should
brush the insides of your knees as you lower. Try to get your thighs lower than parallel
with the floor. Push through your heels to raise yourself back to the starting position.
That's 1 rep. Do 8 to 12.

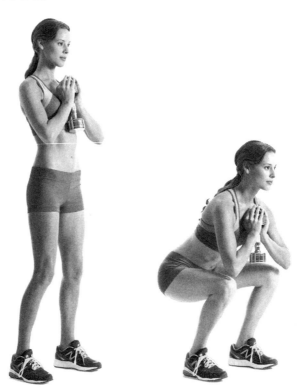

Energy Peanuts

When you're tired and need a lift, pass on the
coffee or those expensive caffeinated multihour
energy shots and have a club soda with lime.
The carbonation and aroma will energize you.

HAMMER CURL
TO PRESS

MUSCLES WORKED
Biceps and shoulders

STARTING POSITION

Hold a pair of dumbbells at your sides, palms facing in (neutral grip), feet hip width apart.

THE MOVE

Curl the weights to your shoulders, then press them overhead until your arms are straight and the weights are directly over your shoulders. Slowly reverse the movement to return to the starting position. That's 1 rep. Do 8 to 12.

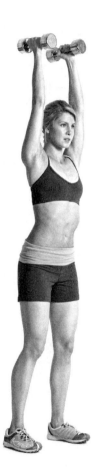
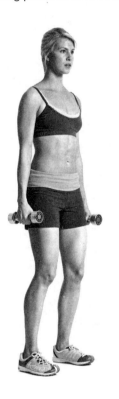
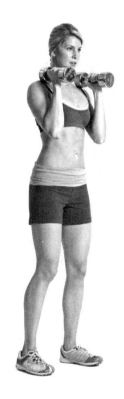

DUMBBELL DEADLIFT

STARTING POSITION

Hold a pair of dumbbells in front of your thighs with your feet hip width apart and your knees slightly bent. Maintain an arch in your back throughout the exercise.

THE MOVE

Bend from your hips to lower your torso until it's almost parallel to the floor, keeping the weights close to your body. Return to standing. That's 1 rep. Do 8 to 12.

FIT TIP

When lowering and rising, it's crucial to keep the weights close to your body, as if you're shaving your legs with them, to prevent straining your back.

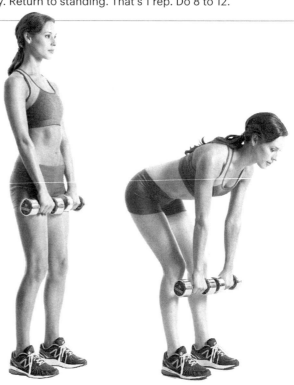

Energy Peanuts

Carry essential oils. Smelling peppermint can boost exercise performance. Researchers say that the scent of mint alters your perception of how hard you're exercising, which can make workouts seem less strenuous so you don't mind exercising longer.

SINGLE-ARM DUMBBELL ROW AND TWIST

MUSCLES WORKED
Upper back and core

STARTING POSITION

Hold a dumbbell in your right hand, bend at your hips and knees, and lower your torso until it's about 45 degrees to the floor. Let the dumbbell hang at arm's length from your shoulder, palm facing in.

THE MOVE

In one motion, pull the dumbbell toward your body while rotating your torso to the right, keeping your elbow tucked close to your side. Pause, then lower the weight back to the starting position. That's 1 rep. Complete 10 reps, then repeat on the other side.

FIT TIP

Do this exercise slowly to focus on proper form. Once you get the hang of it, you can speed up. Also, consider placing your nonworking hand on a bench or chair for stability.

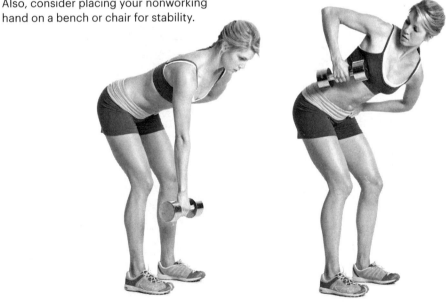

DUMBBELL PULLOVER

STARTING POSITION

Lie faceup on a flat bench with only your head and upper
back on the pad. Hold the weights directly over your
chest with your feet flat on the floor.

THE MOVE

Without changing the angle of your elbows, slowly lower the dumbbells back beyond
your head until your upper arms are in line with your body and parallel to the floor.
Pause, then slowly raise the dumbbells back to the starting position. That's 1 rep.
Do 8 to 12.

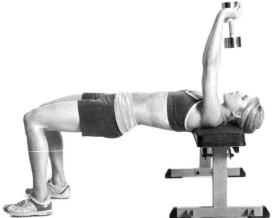

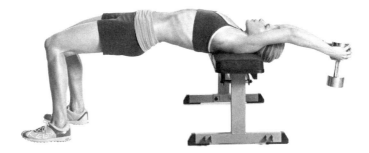

Energy Peanuts

Studies show that listening to
your favorite music while
exercising can boost your
endurance by 15 percent.

Phase 3

45 MINUTES

THE FAT-BURNER SUPERSET

You will tone your muscles, build agility, and improve balance and reaction time with this challenging Phase 3 workout. But best of all, the built-in jumps will fire up your metabolism for greater fat burn. You will need two 8- to 12-pound dumbbells or an 18-pound body bar for this workout. The eight exercises shown on the following pages will be done in superset style. In other words, you will perform each pair of exercises back-to-back without rest in between. After completing the second move in the pair, you'll rest for up to 2 minutes before starting the second superset and so on. After the fourth superset, rest 2 minutes and repeat supersets 1 through 4. Before you begin, warm up your muscles with 5 minutes of brisk walking or rope jumping.

Superset 1

CLEAN AND PRESS

MUSCLES WORKED
Back, shoulders, arms, glutes, and hamstrings

STARTING POSITION

Stand with your feet shoulder width apart and knees bent to 45 degrees. Hold a pair of dumbbells at your sides with your palms facing you.

THE MOVE

Quickly pull your hands up to shoulder height, palms facing forward, while simultaneously straightening your legs to stand upright. When the weights reach shoulder height, drop your elbows beside your ribs, bend your legs slightly, then press your hands overhead while straightening your legs. Return your hands to shoulder height, then slide them down your thighs and bend your knees to return to start. Do 8 to 10 reps.

FIT TIP

Be sure to bend your knees slightly after cleaning the dumbbells to your shoulders to load your legs so your hamstrings can help you move the dumbbells overhead when you straighten your legs.

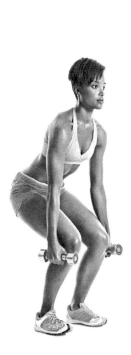
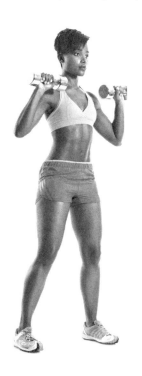
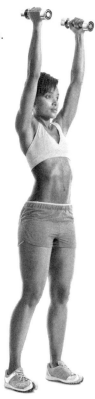

POWER SQUAT

STARTING POSITION

Standing with your feet shoulder width apart, hold a body bar or barbell behind your shoulders (or hold a pair of dumbbells at your shoulders).

THE MOVE

Sit your butt back as if sitting in a chair, taking 3 seconds to squat, until your hips are level with your knees. Straighten your legs to return to standing as quickly as you can. That's 1 rep. Do 10.

Rest for 2 minutes.

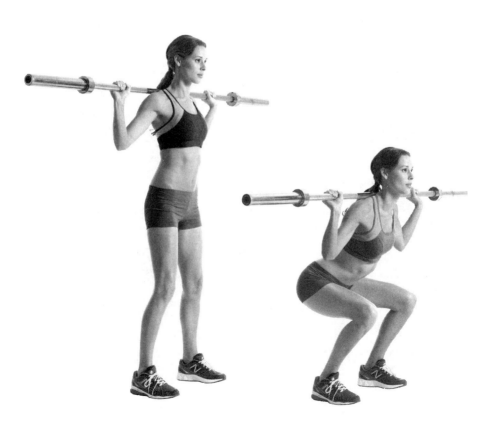

Superset 2

CURTSY LUNGE

MUSCLES WORKED
Glutes, hips, quadriceps, hamstrings

STARTING POSITION

Stand with your feet hip width apart, hands holding dumbbells at your sides.

THE MOVE

Take a big step back with your right leg, crossing it behind your left. Bend your knees and lower your hips until your left thigh is nearly parallel to the floor. Keep your torso upright and your hips and shoulders as square as possible. Return to the starting position. Perform 8 to 10 reps, and then repeat, stepping back with your left leg for 8 to 10 reps. Add dumbbells once you master the movement with perfect form.

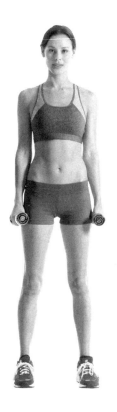

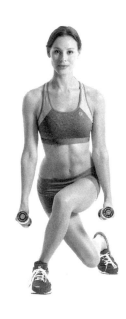

LATERAL LUNGE

STARTING POSITION

Standing with your feet hip-width apart, hold a pair of dumbbells, palms facing in.

THE MOVE

Take a step to the left, transferring all your weight onto your left leg, and sink into a lunge while your hands, holding the dumbbells, drop toward the floor. Don't round your back; keep a natural arch in your lower back as you lower. Return to standing as you step your left foot next to the right. Pause, then repeat to the other side, stepping with your right foot. Do 8 to 10 reps on each side.

Rest for 2 minutes.

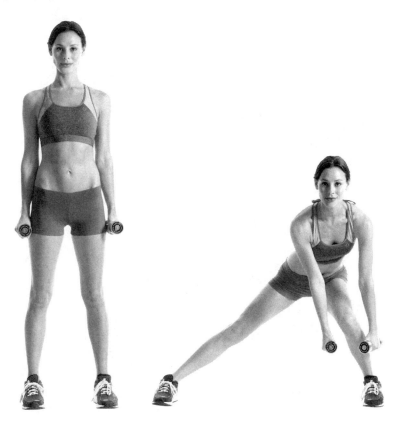

YOGA PUSHUP

MUSCLES WORKED
Chest, arms, and car-diovascular system

STARTING POSITION

Get in a pushup position with your hands directly under your shoulders.

THE MOVE

Bend your elbows to lower your chest toward the floor. Then straighten your arms and as you return to the start, raise your hips up in the air while driving your heels into the ground. You'll end up in a downward-facing dog yoga position. Reset to the starting position. That's 1 rep. Do 8 to 10.

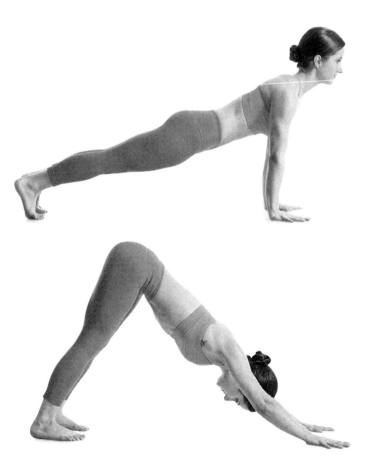

BENCH PRESS

MUSCLES WORKED
Chest and arms

STARTING POSITION

Lie faceup on an exercise bench, feet flat on the floor.
Hold dumbbells with your hands shoulder width apart, the weights at your chest, elbows bent out to the sides. Your palms should face your feet.

THE MOVE

Slowly press the weights upward until your arms are straight and your hands are above your chest. Return to the starting position. Do 8 to 10 reps.

Rest for 2 minutes.

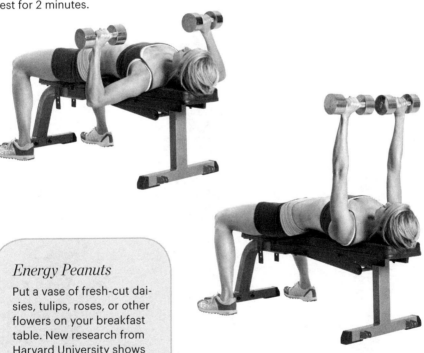

Energy Peanuts

Put a vase of fresh-cut dai-sies, tulips, roses, or other flowers on your breakfast table. New research from Harvard University shows that even people who say they're not "morning peo-ple" report feeling happier and more energetic after looking at flowers first thing in the a.m.

Superset 4

JUMP POWER LUNGE

MUSCLES WORKED
Quadriceps, glutes, calves, hamstrings, and cardiovascular system

STARTING POSITION

Without using dumbbells, stand in a staggered lunge position with your left leg forward and bent at 90 degrees and right leg back, knee hovering about an inch over the floor. Keep your hands on your hips and your chest up.

THE MOVE

Explosively press your feet into the floor to jump straight up. At the peak of the jump, switch leg positions in midair so that you land with your legs in opposite positions. Land and dip into the lunge and immediately repeat. Do 20 jumps.

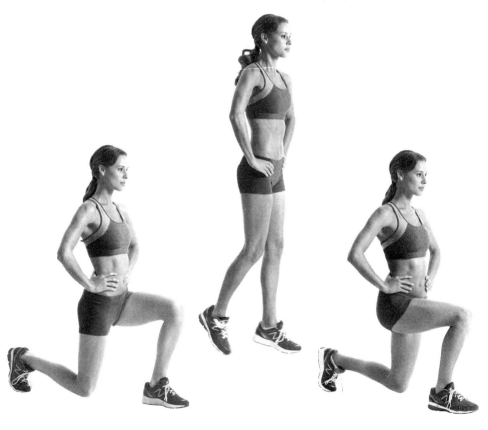

DOUBLE REVERSE LUNGE

MUSCLES WORKED
Quadriceps and calves

STARTING POSITION

Stand with your feet together, holding dumbbells at your sides, palms facing in.

THE MOVE

Take a step backward with your right leg until your knee hovers an inch above the ground. Keep your spine straight as you lean slightly forward, then press through your left foot to push back to standing. Repeat on the left side. Do 10 reps per leg.

Rest for 2 minutes.

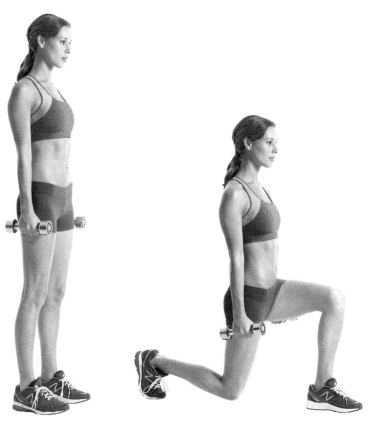

25 MINUTES

ON AND OFF

This HIIT running workout is super easy to remember. You'll see in a sec. It's also super efficient. In one study, participants who followed a similar program three times a week for 2 weeks saw the same benefits as those who completed 10 hours of moderate exercise during the 2 weeks. Add one On and Off workout to your Phase 3 schedule. You'll need a sports watch for this program.

WARMUP: Jog or do jumping jacks or other dynamic calisthenics or jump rope for 3 to 5 minutes.

ON: Sprint. For 30 seconds, run at a pace that leaves you winded but not breathless. (Think 8 out of 10, with 10 being your top speed.)

OFF: Recover! For 1 minute, jog or walk. (You should be able to carry on a conversation by the end.)

Repeat the pattern 10 times, then finish with a 3- to 5-minute cooldown.

YOGA IN A FLASH

Just 5 to 10 minutes of yoga can make a difference to your mind and body, says Kathryn Budig, author of *The Women's Health Big Book of Yoga*. "The trick is to set an intention each time you roll out your mat," she says. "Before you start moving, decide how you want to feel after your practice—more relaxed, energized, or stronger—then keep your intention in mind as you move." These quick tips will help get you even closer to your goal.

Energize: Increase your heart rate by moving rapidly through five Sun Salutations.

Stretch: Anytime you do Downward-Facing Dog or Forward Fold, hold for five deep breaths.

Strengthen: Do Warrior 2 or Crescent poses. Hold lunging poses for at least 60 seconds, focusing on lowering deeper and deeper into the posture.

Calm: End in Corpse pose with 1 to 3 minutes of silence and stillness; as you lie there, breathe deeply and imagine your body sinking into the floor.

SUN SALUTATION

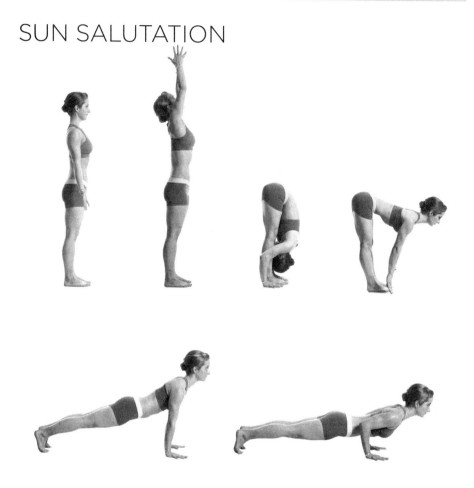

MOUNTAIN: Stand tall, arms at your sides, palms facing out. Keep your shoulders down and push your tailbone toward your heels.

MOUNTAIN WITH ARMS OVERHEAD: Inhale as you raise your arms straight up and join your palms. Relax the base of your neck and keep your quads lifted.

STANDING FORWARD FOLD: Exhale as you extend forward from your hips, straighten your legs, and fold forward to the floor. Keep your hips stacked over your heels and elongate your core.

HALF-STANDING FORWARD FOLD: Inhale as you keep your hands down and extend your chest and gaze.

PLANK: Exhale, place your palms flat on the floor, and step your feet back into a plank. Your shoulders should be directly over your wrists. Keep your core engaged. Reach your tailbone toward your heels.

PUSHUP: Bend your elbows to lower your body into a pushup position. Keep your elbows in toward your ribs. Engage your quads.

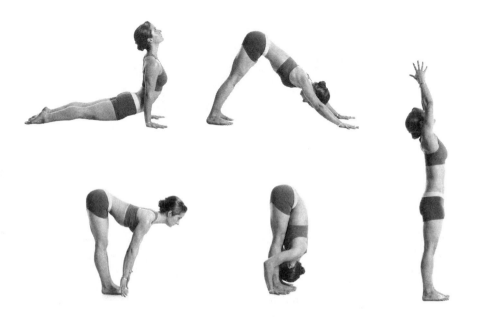

UPWARD-FACING DOG: Inhale as you roll over your toes, and press away from the floor to lift your chest. Roll your shoulders back.

DOWNWARD-FACING DOG: Exhale, then roll your toes back over as you lift and press your hips back. Take five breaths in this position. Be sure to draw your ribs in toward your spine. Your upper body should form a straight line from fingertips to tailbone.

HALF-STANDING FORWARD FOLD: Inhale and gaze forward as you lengthen back into your legs and bend your knees. Exhale, and step or jump forward to meet your hands. Inhale as you extend your gaze and chest.

STANDING FORWARD FOLD: Exhale as you fold forward over your legs. Keep your shoulders lifted away from your ears.

MOUNTAIN WITH ARMS OVERHEAD: Inhale as you extend your arms to the sides. Lift your chest, come all the way up to standing, and press your palms overhead, keeping your arms straight. End in Mountain: Exhale as you release your arms and lower them next to your body.

DOWNWARD-FACING DOG

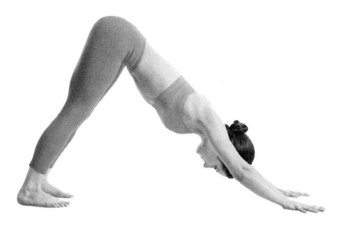

From a pushup position with your arms and legs fully extended (wrists directly under your shoulders), contract your core and abdominal muscles. Slowly exhale and shift your weight backward by pushing your hips up and back. Continue moving until your body forms an inverted V, allowing your head to hang loosely between your shoulders. Keep your arms and legs extended, and be sure to maintain a neutral (flat) spine. Hold for 1 minute.

WARRIOR 2

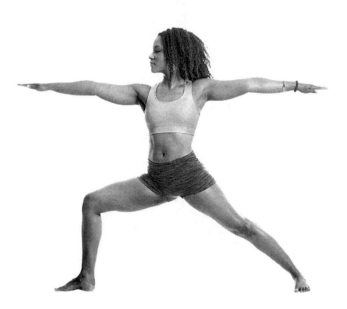

Start with your feet parallel and one leg length apart. Rotate your left foot out 90 degrees and your right foot in slightly, so your left heel is lined up with your right foot's arch. Bend your front knee, bringing your thigh parallel to the floor with your knee over your heel. Keep your torso directly over your pelvis. Relax your lower back and keep your front ribs in. Keeping your inner elbows straight, reach actively with your arms to raise them parallel to the floor. Gaze over your front fingertips. Repeat on the other side.

CRESCENT

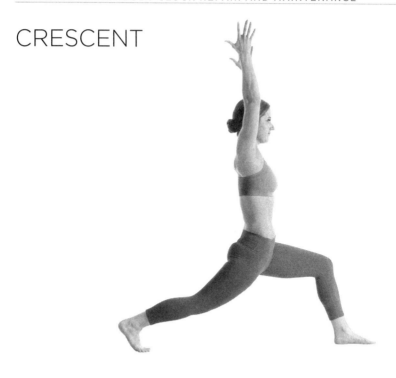

Start in Mountain pose (page 220), then step back about one leg length with your right foot as you bend your left knee 90 degrees. Keep both feet hip width apart, with your weight resting on the heel of your front foot and on the ball of your back foot. Engage your lower belly to extend your lower back. Raise your arms straight over your head. Rotate your upper arms inward and lift your gaze. Keep your hips level. Repeat on the opposite side.

Energy Peanuts

Leave your running shoes by the front door. Put a water bottle you got at a fitness event on your work desk. The more closely you associate exercise with your personal identity, the more likely you are to make sweating part of your daily routine, according to an international team of US and Canadian scientists.

CORPSE

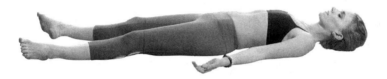

Lie on your back. Spread your arms a comfortable distance away from your body. Turn your palms up. Move your legs a natural distance apart. Relax your feet and allow them to roll outward. Close your eyes.

Energy Peanuts

Stretch like a cat for 30 to 60 seconds when you roll out of bed each morning. It's like hitting a reset button on your body. Get on all fours on the floor and curl your back toward the ceiling like a frightened cat. Hold for 10 seconds, then bend in the opposite direction, lowering your belly button toward the floor while keeping your arms straight, hands directly under your shoulders and thighs perpendicular to the floor. Catlike stretching first thing in the morning improves posture, promotes bloodflow, and relieves body tension, according to the *Big Book of Uncommon Knowledge* by the editors of *Men's Health*.

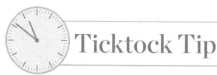

Ticktock Tip

What's the Best Time of Day to Exercise?

Morning. Also midmorning and noon. Two p.m. is fine, and 5 p.m. is really good.

Seriously, any exercise at any time is better than none. And according to research on mice from the University of California, Los Angeles's Brain Research Institute, exercising anytime during the daylight hours can improve your sleep and reduce your risk for health problems associated with a disrupted internal clock, such as weight gain, cardiovascular disease, and immune system dysfunction.

One thing to consider: Your core temperature is lower in the morning, so if you work out at that time, make sure you warm up properly before jumping into rigorous exercise. Your body tends to be warmer in the late afternoon and evening, which corresponds with greater performance, researchers say. What about exercising at night? It really depends how late you're planning. A recent study by the National Sleep Foundation found that, compared to non-exercisers, people who work out are more likely to say they sleep well no matter when they broke a sweat. But remember that your internal body temperature cools at the end of the day to make you sleepy. A big sweat session at 10:00 or 11:00 will likely affect your sleep and throw off your body clock.

HOW TO EAT BEFORE EXERCISE

If you plan to exercise for 45 minutes or less and you've eaten a nutritious meal within the last 2, even 3 hours, there's no reason you need a pre-workout snack.

However, if you haven't eaten, you'll want to energize your workout. Just make it appropriate for the intensity of the exercise. This chart will help.

Activity	Combo Snack	Why
Walking	Pear + ½ oz cheese	Low-intensity exercise requires a light snack. Keep it around 100 calories.
Yoga	1 cup low-fat milk + 2 oz turkey	To avoid bloating when trying to do Downward-Facing Dog, grab a snack of 200 calories of easily digested carbs and protein. Eat at least 1 hour before your class.
Strength training	1 cup Greek yogurt + 1 medium banana	Shoot for 250 calories' worth of muscle-building protein and energizing carbs at least 30 minutes prior to lifting and you'll jump-start recovery.
Running	½ whole-wheat bagel + 1 Tbsp almond butter	Heavy foods will slow you down and slosh around. Aim for 300 calories of roughly 30 g carbs for fast-burning energy no later than an hour before your run.

CHAPTER
14

The Mommy Clock

HOW TO INGRAIN YOUR ENTIRE FAMILY WITH THE PRINCIPLES OF POSITIVE NUTRITION

Here at *Women's Health*, we're well aware that being a mom is a full-time job. In fact, if you have a career outside the house, you're really working two full-time jobs, and that can be an extra strain on the rhythm of your body clock. I know. I'm a 40-year-old full-time dietitian/nutritionist and mother of two boys. I know how challenging the daily responsibility of feeding a family can be. It's even more daunting when you consider that it's your responsibility (and your partner's if you have one) to raise your kids to love eating all foods, to respect and love their body shapes, and to establish other healthy habits such as exercise.

How do you do it? You already have the tools. I encourage you to teach your child or children the Five Pillars of Positive Nutrition and to practice the self-care and self-compassion strategies you have learned through *The Women's Health Body Clock Diet*.

As you work your way through the 6 weeks of the program's lifestyle prep, feel free to feed your family the same meals. All children need the same three macronutrients—carbohydrates, proteins, and fats—that you do. Preplanned snacks with two of the three macronutrients are a must for your children; we aren't talking about grazing. Rather, children need meal and snack times consistent with the daily meal structure of the Body Clock Diet. All the foods suggested in this book are appropriate for the entire family.

RAISING A MINDFUL EATER

We all live in a weight-obsessed society, and it's our job to make food peace for our children and ourselves. In my early thirties, I had my firstborn son, Robert. I was determined that he would grow up in a neutral food environment, that is, a home that didn't label foods good or bad, a home without the clean plate club, and a home that emphasized internal self-regulation. Most children are adept at self-regulation, what I call the "honor system" in this book. It's parents and grandparents and our food-and-weight-obsessed culture that introduce children to fad dieting, a messed-up hunger/fullness cycle, and body bashing. But my son is proof that with the right approach, like All Foods Fit and others encouraged in this book, kids can be protected from eating disorders and unhealthy weight.

While my son is definitely a picky eater, he's most secure in his ability to read his internal biological system that's synchronized with circadian rhythm. He knows what hunger and fullness feel like. He can eat two bites of ice cream and be full. He knows he can save the rest for another day. Sometimes I open his lunch box and wonder why he left something. He tells me, "I wanted to eat something else and save that for a snack after school." He is in tune with his mind and body. He is an expert at getting up from the table, checking his belly-brain connection, and coming back to his meal when he's hungry again. He tells adults that he doesn't need to clean his plate. He explains to his friends that pizza is not bad. Pizza has carbohydrates, proteins, and fats. You can offer him ice cream or pizza and he'll say "No, thank you" if he isn't hungry, because he knows he can have it later or the next day. We leave our Halloween candy out and our gingerbread houses at eye level. He's not out of control in this environment, and typically he forgets that these sugary temptations are there. Do I sound like a proud mom? Well, I am. But I'm not any different from you, even though I have a dietitian's degree and a certain expertise. All I did was allow my child to follow his natural feeding and eating practices, driven by his circadian rhythm. I didn't interfere but only gently guided.

Obviously our environment teaches us something else. Our culture focuses on external practices such as measuring, counting calories and points, and restricting whole food groups. Skipping meals is wrongly thought of as willpower. We all have to contend with societal messages and peer pressure. You can help change this for yourself, for your kids, and for others. You have likely already reset your clock so you can work with internal regulation. Once you master this, please remember that this is a lifestyle, and you can pay it forward by teaching others to turn inward and honor their minds and bodies and not abuse or ignore them.

ROUND-THE-CLOCK SNACKS FOR KIDS

Let children use their hunger fullness cues to determine their portions. Notice that the following snacks contain at least two of the three macronutrients.

Morning snack ideas

- Homemade Yummy Tummy Blueberry Muffins and a warm pat of natural butter (see recipe on page 232).

- Fresh berries with sliced real cheese (not processed cheese product)

- Greek yogurt (the adult version, not the kids' style sweetened with tons of added sugar) with 2 teaspoons wheat germ

- Clif Kid Z bar with a glass of milk

Midday snack ideas

- Hummus and whole wheat pita

- Blue corn chips with fresh salsa and black pitted olives

- About 2 cookies with a glass of milk

- Dried fruit (no added sugar or preservatives) and sunflower butter

- Frozen banana with almond butter

Yummy Tummy Blueberry Muffins

This is a wonderful warm snack to share with your child. I've included no nutrition facts for this recipe because it's designed to be a cooking experience for bonding with your child and practicing enjoying the muffin using your five senses and hunger/fullness cues.

Make this recipe with your youngster to model the All Foods Fit concept and the act of self-care through cooking.

Yields 12 muffins

½ cup whole wheat flour

1 cup white flour

1 cup oats (old-fashioned, uncooked)

½ cup + 6 teaspoons sugar

1 tablespoon baking powder

1 cup unsweetened organic almond, soy, or regular milk

¼ cup GMO-free canola oil

1 egg, lightly beaten

2 teaspoons pure vanilla extract

1 cup fresh blueberries, washed (organic, if possible)

6 teaspoons cinnamon

1. Preheat the oven to 400°F. Coat 2 muffin tins with GMO-free canola oil spray.

2. In a large bowl, combine the wheat flour, white flour, oats, ½ cup sugar, and baking powder. Mix well. In a separate bowl, combine the milk, oil, egg, and vanilla. Blend well. Add the liquid mixture to the dry ingredients and mix until the batter is moist and the ingredients are blended. Gently stir in the blueberries.

3. Fill the muffin cups three-quarters full. Bake for 15 to 20 minutes.

4. Meanwhile, in a small bowl, combine the 6 teaspoons sugar and cinnamon.

5. The muffins are ready when the edges start to pull away from the muffin pan and/or when a toothpick inserted in the center of a muffin comes out clean (no batter) upon removal. Cool the muffins in the pan on a wire rack for about 5 minutes. Sprinkle with the sugar and cinnamon, remove from the muffin pan, and serve with a fresh slab of butter.

Evening snack ideas

- Frozen Greek yogurt squeezer (I recommend Siggi's, Stonyfield Farms, and Horizon's versions) with a side of fresh fruit

- Ice cream or sorbet: Yes, the real thing! Think Häagen-Dazs or a local purveyor.

- Apples and natural peanut butter (nothing but peanuts and salt on the ingredients list)

- Carrots and ranch dressing

ALLOW ALL FOODS; DON'T SWEAT IT

Focus on providing your family with wholesome and less-processed foods the majority of the time and low-nutrient foods some of the time. This allows for flexibility in food choices and will prevent your child from becoming a restrained eater. Following the All Foods Fit philosophy, you can allow two "sometimes foods," that is, low-nutrient snacks, every day or even one fast-food meal. The point is, don't sweat the small stuff. Focus on how you feed the family at home and allow all foods. If your child is hiding food or you find snack wrappers under his bed, he already feels restricted. Don't worry. Just monitor your food language around him and be aware of how you talk about your own body. Be very careful about using the word *diet*. Below I've listed some examples of what many of us may say mindlessly and may be misinterpreted by a child, as well as some gentler words you may want to use instead.

What-Not-to-Say Cheat Sheet

Moms, use this What-Not-to-Say Cheat Sheet to help guide your word choices when speaking to your children and, of course, to yourself!

DON'T SAY: "OMG, you lost so much weight! What are your secrets?"

DO SAY: "How are you doing? It's so good to see you."

DON'T SAY: "Oh, honey, you could stand to lose a few pounds."

DO SAY: "Are you eating for fuel? Are you bored or maybe even sad?"

DON'T SAY: "If you don't lose weight, you're never going to have friends or get a good job!"

DO SAY: "Your body size does not dictate your success or self-worth."

DON'T SAY: "Candy is junk food and bad."

DO SAY: "How do you feel after eating candy? Does it keep you energized and full for a long time? "

DON'T SAY: "You need to exercise or you'll get fat."

DO SAY: "Move your body to keep it strong and give yourself rest time too."

DON'T SAY: "You need to eat your veggies because they're good for you."

DO SAY: "Let's try to eat veggies every day to get the necessary vitamins our bodies and minds need. Maybe we can use a star chart to help you try new kinds of vegetables."

DON'T SAY: "That's bad for you. You ate so much junk food today."

DO SAY: "Let's think about what you ate today. Did you meet your nutrition needs to grow?"

REDEFINE *DIET*

As you move through the phases of the Body Clock Diet, it's important to redefine the word *diet* for your children, especially if they see you reading this book with the word on the cover. Use the definition found in *Webster's Dictionary*, "habitual nourishment." The goal is to neutralize the word *diet* so it carries no special meaning. A diet is simply what we eat every day. Stop thinking of *diet* as a short-term crash or fad diet for the purpose of losing weight quickly while restricting eating. The goal is to prevent eating disorders and disordered eating while achieving a state of optimal wellness mentally and physically. Wellness is the goal of your family; everyone's weight will be a result of the wellness.

REDIRECT CONVERSATION

If you see a girlfriend while you're out and about and she says, "OMG, you look amazing! You've lost weight. What diet are you on?" you can reply, "Hi, how are you? We are super well. And oh, we've simply made lifestyle changes based on our 24-hour body clock. It's really about habitual nourishment. We're eating wholesome foods the majority of the time and regularly while also honoring our hunger and fullness cues. It's a whole self-care routine." (Then loan her a copy of *The Women's Health Body Clock Diet*!)

Your answer signifies that asking "how someone is" will always be first priority. The number of pounds someone may have lost is irrelevant. Rather, your beautiful glow and big smile are the clues revealing you've changed your lifestyle with a self-care routine and reset your body clock. Using the words *lifestyle* and *self-care routine* suggests this isn't a crash diet your friend may have been alluding to. Meanwhile, your child interprets it as "resetting your body's clock and changing the family's habitual nourishment." I mean, by this point the child knows the real definition of diet is "habitual nourishment."

PROTECT YOUR KIDS FROM BMI LABELING

Early in the book, we talked briefly about body mass index, also known as BMI. Perhaps your own medical doctor has said your BMI is too high and you have to lose weight. As I stressed before, BMI is an inaccurate measure of health and fitness for adults and for children as well. A higher BMI doesn't mean you have to lose weight, as it's based on scale weight. In addition, adult BMIs greater than 35 or less than 18.5 are the only categories associated with greater mortality. Don't get caught up in the numbers game with BMIs or the scale for you or your child. Focusing on the numbers is likely to cause you to restrict certain foods for your child or for your child to become a restrained eater. This is not desirable; the famed Framingham Heart Study showed that weight cycling (aka yo-yoing) as a result of restrictive dieting is associated with higher mortality and cardiac disease. It's actually healthier to be at a higher set weight than to allow your weight to fluctuate up and down by 20 pounds. You are your child's role model. Be wary of BMI labels for both adults and children and never put yourself or your child on a "start/stop" fad diet.

Children's BMI Screening in School

Be aware that BMI labeling is now being used in certain school districts by school nurses as a measurement to screen children for obesity. This is controversial due to the fact that only one governing health agency, the Institute of Medicine, recommends BMI screening for children in schools. Other agencies, including the Centers for Disease Control, the US Preventive Services Task Force, and the American Academy of Pediatrics, do not endorse school screening for BMI. Why? Because no research supports the effectiveness of identifying BMI in school-age children. If you live in New York, Arkansas, or California, expect that your child will be screened and will likely bring home a BMI report card. I'm very concerned that focusing on weight, especially by use of this tool, rather than promoting overall health for children will increase their chances of body dissatisfaction, body shaming, and, ultimately, eating disorders. And you should be, too.

If your child comes home one day with a "BMI report card," also known as a FitnessGram, don't worry and please don't make a big deal of it in front of your child. Focus instead on providing the body clock meal structure of three meals and two or three snacks daily (depending on age, level of activity, and the child's needs). Your goal should be a child with a healthy mind, body, and spirit, no matter her BMI or weight. If you are concerned, seek the guidance of a pediatrician and a registered dietitian specializing in eating disorders, as they will be sensitive to food language and the All Foods Fit concept to help you and your child embrace lifestyle changes, not calorie restrictions.

HELPING WITH THE HUNGER DIALOGUE

Your child's food intake, just like yours, doesn't need to be perfect. One of the more important concepts to teach your child is honoring her body in all ways by recognizing hunger and fullness. Most babies are born able to initiate and disengage from feeding. I encourage you to dialogue with your child about hunger and fullness. Help her to respect her body and understand what messages her body is conveying. Here are five questions to help your child focus inward.

Hunger Talk

- "What foods keep you full the longest?"

- "Did you eat enough to keep you full until lunchtime?"

- "Why do you think you're emotional today?" (Perhaps she didn't eat lunch at school, and the child can associate extreme hunger with becoming emotional.)

- "Are you hungry for a snack or do you want it a little later?"

- "Are you full? If you are, you can save your dessert for tomorrow."

> ## Four Coping Skills for Children
>
> Body scan (as taught in Chapter 8)
>
> Four-pebble meditation (see below)
>
> Feelings talk
>
> Creating art

You're providing the kids with meals and snacks, but they'll determine portions under your guidance. Again, don't be rigid and don't strive for perfection. Teach your child resiliency and coping skills before he develops emotional and behavioral relationships with food.

One of my favorite tools to use with my 8-year-old son is the body scan you learned in Chapter 8. If he can't fall asleep, we lie together and I lead him in the body scan, starting with his toes and ending with his head. He tells me, "It's so relaxing." Music to my ears, and it will be for you too.

Thich Nhat Hanh, the Zen teacher we referred to earlier in the book, has written children's books. The one titled *A Handful of Quiet: Happiness in Four Pebbles* is a great introduction to meditation for children. While these techniques are basically similar to your new skills, children need to learn their own versions.

Teaching children to talk about their feelings and the act of validating these feelings are extremely important. Keep in mind that you may have to first help them put words to their feelings. Todd Parr's *The Feelings Book* and online resources such as "Teaching Your Child to Identify and Express Emotions" from Vanderbilt University are great tools to start this conversation.

Children are awesome artists. Allow them to express their feelings through different media as another avenue to express emotions. Finger painting, molding mud, drawing, and coloring are all easy forms of art to release emotions.

BUILDING RESILIENCE

Resilience is the ability to adapt well to adversity, trauma, tragedy, threats, or even significant sources of stress. It's an important skill to master, and it can help your children manage stress and feelings of anxiety and uncertainty. Here are steps to help you help your kids develop resilience. They are adapted from "The Road to Resilience" from the American Psychological Association and enhanced for the Body Clock Diet lifestyle. (Italics are my additions.)

1. **Make connections.** Teach your child how to make friends, including the skill of empathy, or feeling another's pain.

2. **Help your child by having her help others.** Children who may feel helpless can be empowered by helping others.

3. **Maintain a daily routine.** Sticking to a routine can be comforting to children, especially younger children who crave structure in their lives. Encourage your child to develop his own routines.

   Think about this as something similar to your resetting your body clock. Structure is important for you and your children mentally and physically.

4. **Take a break.** While it's important to stick to routines, endless worrying can be counterproductive. Teach your child how to focus on something besides what's worrying him. This is in line with the Body Clock Diet lifestyle that stresses flexibility and the need to decrease stress.

5. **Teach your child self-care.** Make yourself a good example and teach your child the importance of making time to eat, exercise, and rest. Make sure your child has time to have fun and you haven't scheduled every moment of her life with no downtime to relax. Self-care and even having fun will help your child stay balanced and deal better with stressful times. Meal structure, mindfulness, and meditating are key in both your life and your child's.

6. **Move toward your goals.** Teach your child to set reasonable goals and then to move toward them one step at a time.

   Baby steps, realistic small steps, working in phases, or whatever way you identify it—understanding the process of achieving a goal is as important as eventually achieving the goal.

7. **Nurture a positive self-view.** Help your child remember ways that she has handled hardships in the past and then help her understand that these tough times help build the strength to handle future challenges.

8. **Keep things in perspective and maintain a hopeful outlook.** Even when your child faces very painful events, help him look at the situation in a broader context and keep a long-term perspective. Although your child may be too young to consider a long-term view on his own, help him see that there's a future beyond the current situation and the future can be good.

   This concept is similar to body acceptance and weight loss. You may not see immediate changes in your body, but better behaviors will result in better health. Teach your child to focus on health for an energized mind and body, not weight reasons.

9. **Look for opportunities for self-discovery.** Tough times are often the times when children learn the most about themselves.

   Your transformation of self-growth and wellness will provide your children with the example of self-discovery that will then help them in their own process as they grow up.

10. **Accept that change is part of living.** Change often can be scary for children and teens. Help your child see that change is part of life and new goals can replace goals that have become unattainable.

    Again, your journey of self-care and self-compassion will lend itself to building resiliency in your children. You are their role model. Lead by example; don't preach. Or act on what you preach.

For more information on raising children with a positive nutrition philosophy, join me and other mommy RDs as we share our wisdom, trials, and tribulations at LauraCipullo.com and MomDishesItOut.com. I also recommend two must-reads for every new mom: *Child of Mine: Feeding with Love and Good Sense,* by Ellyn Satter, RD, and *Happy Mealtimes with Happy Kids: How to Teach Your Child about the Joy of Food,* by Melanie Potock.

Special Section

A FINAL MESSAGE,
PLUS STORIES OF SUCCESS

Thank you for joining me on this journey toward wellness. I'm certain that if you've followed the advice in this book and reset your faulty master body clock, you're feeling better physically and mentally. You're nourishing your body properly—eating all foods, even cookies for snacks—sleeping better, exercising with energy and enthusiasm, and being mindful about managing the stresses in your life. The benefit of all this will be a healthier body in rhythm and, consequently, natural weight loss.

But the journey doesn't end here. Unlike fad diets that have an endpoint when the sacrifice stops, the Body Clock Diet is a program that endures because it's about establishing rhythms and habits that last a lifetime. And by now you have the knowledge and skills to reset your master clock anytime it's running off schedule to ensure good health and a healthy mind, body, and spirit for life.

To review, these are the habits and skills we've learned through the Body Clock Diet program.

1. Start each morning with a mug of hot water.

2. Never starve yourself, and always eat enough to maintain a high metabolism, which we nutritionists call optimal thermogenesis.

3. Enjoy eating all foods, even cookies and french fries.

4. Enjoy one to two glasses of wine weekly if you were a wine drinker before the program.

5. Read through the Five Pillars of Positive Nutrition until they are ingrained.

6. Reduce the effect of the stress response using Cortisol Crushers like relaxation breathing, self-compassion, mindfulness, and meditation.

7. Synchronize circadian rhythm through sleep habituation.

8. Synchronize circadian rhythm using the body clock meal structure and incorporate internal self-awareness to recognize hunger/fullness cues.

9. Recognize the impact of stress on weight and your immune system.

10. Understand that elevated cortisol can be reduced by self-compassion and cuddling with a loved one.

11. Identify feelings, thoughts, and behaviors around food and how they affect your hunger, your weight, and your mental health.

12. Practice mindful eating daily.

13. Practice mindfulness and self-compassion daily.

14. Devote a time of day to you and your self-care.

These simple habits have helped me and hundreds of my clients to reset our body clocks and overcome the behaviors that contribute to overeating, weight gain, and poor health. As you continue on your journey, I hope that the following stories about mindful eating and being will give you inspiration, clarity, and patience during your own transformation. We'll start with my own story of change.

MY NEW RELATIONSHIP WITH FOOD

Looking back at my life long before I became a nutritionist, I realize I was a mindful eater until I entered high school. I was the kid who ate half an apple and left the rest because I was full. I didn't think about when to eat and when to stop,

because it was innate. This changed for me when I was introduced to highly processed foods in seventh and eighth grade. My mom went back to work and my best
friend (who was also a latchkey kid) and I would order ourselves Chinese food,
pizza, or pancakes for school nights. I was quickly developing hedonic hunger. At
school, I wanted to have all the snacks that came in colorful packages, like the ones
my friends brought. As you know, these foods aren't very filling, but they tasted so
good. If I remember correctly, around this time I saw an episode of *Three's Company*. The character Janet was upset. She grabbed a pint of ice cream and began
eating. I don't know why I thought that was a great idea, but it stuck with me. I
still remember sitting in our big den chair, thinking this is what I'm going to do
when I get upset too. Right there, I had a few cracks starting in the mind-body
honor system. This was the beginning of emotional eating.

In the spring of my sophomore year I injured myself playing sports. I could no
longer run or even walk around the block. I kept eating and started gaining a lot of
weight. I was eating behaviorally and even emotionally. It had just become my habit
to eat while studying, to eat when I got home from school, and to eat to avoid my
feelings. I was no longer in touch with my biological need for fuel. This honor system remained broken until I finally learned about the three hungers many years
later in Ellyn Satter's workshop called "Treating the Dieting Casualty." Satter taught
us a "non-diet" approach and "centering" before eating. It changed my life. Happily,
I can say I was able to reharmonize my relationship with food, mind, and body. My
clients and I are real examples of working with your body clock rather than against
it. And you can do it too.

MARY'S STORY

Mindfulness Reveals Emotional Hunger

When my client Mary came to my office for the first time, she feared she
was insatiable. She could never feel full after eating. She had tried her
trainer's high-protein diet and her health coach's gluten-free, dairy-free,
very low-calorie diet. Mary was highly anxious and exercising like a mar-
athon runner. She was bewildered and frustrated by the fact she was
barely eating and overexercising, yet could not lose weight. She hated her

body. Food and body were constantly in her thoughts. At the end of our first session, I asked Mary to do just one thing in the upcoming week: try to identify the hunger type to which she was responding. My intentions were twofold: First, to help her become mindful of why she ate, and second, to connect her with her internal body sensations so she could truly recognize what was driving the intense appetite.

The following week, Mary returned. She reported less hunger. When I asked her what she had learned over the week, she was shocked. By logging her food and feelings, it became evident that she was not eating out of physical hunger; her eating was a behavioral response to feeling anxious. The food helped her numb her anxiety.

In session two, Mary and I created a meal structure to feed her enough fuel to prevent feelings of deprivation. Eating at consistent times throughout the day helped her to prevent bingeing or overeating at night. Over time, Mary learned to turn inward. She became mindful of the three hungers and as a result was able to reduce overeating and better manage her weight.

MOLLY'S STORY

There Are No "Bad" Foods

"The key for me has been getting rid of the food hierarchy. I have realized that by putting all food on the same level, I am really able to enjoy eating. I can finally eat anything I want and not overeat, even the yummiest foods that I had previously deprived myself of. I now know this won't be the last time I have something like french fries. I used to eat every single french fry because I knew they were forbidden and I would not allow them again for a very long time. Now that I put all food on the same level playing field, my eating is different. I allow myself to have what I want. I know there will be a next time and I do not have to gorge on something if I am no longer hungry."

AUBREY'S STORY

All Foods Fit

"In February 2012, I was referred to Laura by my psychologist. We had been working through my weight issues, but my psychologist felt I needed a more encompassing approach. I needed someone who could help with my disordered thinking about food. I needed to gain a greater understanding about nutrition and I needed an individualized plan. My psychologist knew about the nutritionist's 'eating group' and thought it would be beneficial for me to join because it would be a supportive environment. Before my first appointment, I remember thinking, 'I've tried every diet plan (Weight Watchers, Jenny Craig, etc.); why will this be different?' I had no idea that 3 years later, I would have gained much more than I had hoped for. I started with the dinner group, not understanding that my issues with food were more complicated than 'watching what I was eating.' I learned that maybe I was not as hungry as I assumed, that I don't like all fatty 'fun' foods. I learned to taste my food. I used Laura's tools to help me understand what my body was craving.

"After a few months of sessions, Laura added another goal for me: exercise. I hated exercise. I did not want to feel like a failure. Exercise made me think of burning calories. I thought it would only make me feel worse. But Laura arranged a Pilates class for our dinner group and, wow, I ended up enjoying it. I loved our instructor and decided to try individual sessions. It made me feel stronger, and I was forced to accept the way my body looked and to understand that instead of feeling defeated, I needed to feel proud that I was making the effort to take care of myself. After a year of Pilates, Laura suggested I try a spin class. I was scared that I wouldn't be able to finish the session. I was intimidated by the other people who had good bodies, who would be looking at me and judging me for being heavy. But I'm so glad I went. It showed me that I'm capable of pushing myself. Almost 2 years later I am still going to spin class because it makes me feel great.

"I am not scared anymore. I finally feel confident that these new behaviors will never stop. It is my lifestyle. I may not always make the 'better choice,' but I am no longer in denial. I continue to be a work in progress. I haven't binged in over a year! I now allow myself to eat my 'trigger' foods, and these foods no longer have the control over me that they once had."

BECCA'S STORY

Honoring My Internal Scale

"When I first started seeing Laura, I was so frustrated with myself and my body. I had seen multiple nutritionists who preached some version of the same thing: more vegetables and less carbs. There were good foods and bad foods, and I just had to eat more of the good foods and less of the bad foods. I had meal plans created for me. It sounds simple enough. But after years of yo-yo dieting and not being able to stick to these meal plans, I was no better off and felt completely defeated. No matter how hard I tried, it seemed, I could not stick to these plans. I was so frustrated at myself, for gaining the weight in college and not being able to lose it. What was wrong with me? Why could I not lose this weight? I started to wonder if I would ever lose the weight I gained. How could I carry on with all of this negativity toward myself? Would it be like this forever?

"After seeing multiple nutritionists and trying on my own without success, I knew I needed to try something different. Laura's approach was definitely that. When I first started seeing her, I was very skeptical. She told me I needed to start letting myself eat more food, and wanted me to eat the foods I considered 'off-limits' daily. When she worked with me to create my meal plan, I thought she didn't quite understand what I was explaining: that I was trying to *lose* weight. I couldn't imagine how I would eat all of the food that she was telling me to eat, with the big portion sizes, and still lose weight. But she explained that I needed to not be afraid to eat certain foods. She had me keep a food journal, and I kept waiting for her to get mad when she looked and saw I ate more than I 'should' have. But instead she would get excited and tell me I was making progress. Eating ice cream in the middle of the day, just because I want it, is progress?

"Despite my skepticism, I listened to her because my way of losing weight had clearly not worked. So if I wanted cookies, I ate them. If I wanted pasta or pizza, I ate it. Every day I would eat something sweet that I really wanted, just because I wanted it. After a few weeks, maybe a month or so, I would notice that when I went out to dinner and ordered pasta, I wouldn't finish the bowl. I would eat enough to satisfy myself, because I knew that I could have it again if I wanted it. Before, I would have felt so guilty for eating, say, penne with vodka sauce, and then probably would either think the damage was done and eat the whole thing or barely touch it, feel deprived, and then overeat other foods later.

"Laura also told me to stop weighing myself, since I would weigh myself multiple times a day. The number of the scale often dictated my mood, so I threw away my scale. Every week, despite letting myself eat whatever I wanted, I would lose weight. Maybe not as quickly as I would if I had successfully stuck to my meal plan, but not having to focus on the number on the scale allowed me to focus more on how I felt. I focused more on what was I in the mood for and less on what I thought I should eat.

"After a few more months, I started getting comments from people about the weight I had lost. 'What's your secret? Did you cut out carbs?' No, I would respond, I threw away my scale and now let myself eat whatever I want. I say it in a joking way, but it's true. I started seeing Laura about a year and a half ago, and now I can't remember the last time I felt out of control with my eating. I eat when I'm hungry and stop, for the most part, when I'm satisfied. Sometimes I overeat, but it's a conscious choice. I still feel guilty when that happens, but overall I feel so much more comfortable with myself and with my decisions regarding food and exercise. I feel much more free and less judgmental of myself. I used to receive comments about my caloric intake, which would just make me feel worse and self-conscious. But now when I get self-conscious, thinking I'm being watched and judged about my choices, I just remind myself that I'm making this decision consciously. I'm making this decision because it's something I want.

(continued on page 250)

WHEN IT'S NO LONGER A DIET
Know the Signs of an Eating Disorder

What starts as a simple effort to lose weight can become a catastrophe if you aren't careful. Many women start and stop diets and gain and lose weight on a regular basis. What happens when someone doesn't go off a diet? Is it possible that what was once a diet is now an eating disorder? It's important that women know the signs and symptoms of a diet gone awry. Your eating and metabolism can be normalized if you get help.

Take this scenario of a diet gone disordered. Perhaps all the women in your office lost their holiday weight by cutting carbohydrates. Sounds easy enough, so you decide to cut carbs too. Little did you know the other women only reduced their carbohydrates for the initial 2 weeks of their diet. Now, 6 months later, you have continued to restrict carbohydrates, even fruit. Everyone says you look great, and all the guys are commenting on how thin you are. You never miss a day at the gym and have memorized the nutrition labels of every food in your shopping cart. From an outsider's perspective, people think you're super healthy and in control.

However, you feel just the opposite—out of control. You're afraid to eat anything for fear of weight gain. Chicken and broccoli are your safe foods! You have lost weight, but you feel worse now. You have lost your self-esteem. You missed your best friend's birthday dinner to get to your favorite gym class. You stopped drinking alcohol for fear of the extra calories and wouldn't dare to take a bite of the birthday cake.

These feelings and concerns are unhealthy and unnecessary. Women don't need to feel guilty for eating real food. When calorie thoughts consume your day, you know your diet is no longer a diet. Another scenario you may identify with is when your diet becomes a trigger for a binge or an episode of overeating. Perhaps you're counting points for your diet program. However, if you go above your allotted points, you feel like a failure and sabotage yourself. You eat whatever you can. This is not because you're hungry but because you're punishing yourself. You feel out of control with life and your eating. Your refrigerator is your enemy and your friend. The next day you wake up and hate yourself. You vow not to eat for the rest of the day to make up for the extra calories you consumed last night. But you just can't refrain from eating, and you end up ordering Chinese food for dinner and eating a box of cereal for dessert. If you can identify with these thoughts and/or behaviors, your diet is no longer a diet!

Other signs that your eating is becoming disordered include eating the same foods every meal every day; eating only foods with nutrition facts/ labels; refusing to eat/drink the full-fat version of a food if the fat-free version is not available; working out to compensate for the food you ate; restricting food all day in fear of what you may consume at night; feeling out of control in the presence of your "fear" foods; eating food in large quantities despite not feeling hunger; punishing yourself because you "cheated" on your diet; weighing yourself multiple times a day; and feeling sad and moody all day if the scale goes up a pound.

These are just a few examples of signs/symptoms to bring awareness to a possible eating issue. Many women behave in the above manner, but such discomfort with eating and your body is not necessary. You don't fail at diets, rather diets fail you. You can empower change with the right help. Redefine *diet* as habitual nourishment and use the Five Pillars of Positive Nutrition in this book as your daily mantra. If food and body thoughts consume your day, reach out and get help from a professional. Overcome your disordered eating before it becomes an eating disorder. Seek out a registered dietitian and a therapist specializing in eating disorders identified by the initials CEDRD and CEDS (certified eating disorder registered dietitian and certified eating disorder specialist). These professionals have extensive training in helping women and men, adults and children change their relationships to food, body, and self.

Additional resources:

International Association of Eating Disorders Professionals: iaedp.com

National Eating Disorders Association (NEDA): nationaleatingdisorders.org

Binge Eating Disorder Association (BEDA): BEDAonline.com

"Laura has helped me find a plan that works with my schedule and life. With the hours I spend in the office (recently 10 to 12 hours a day, including on weekends), I'm exhausted most of the time. Laura has shown me that it's okay if I can't do everything. She would tell me it's okay if I can't make it to spin, maybe I can get in some walking. But even if I can't get anything in, she would remind me that I have a lot going on right now. She's helped me to stop being so hard on myself, but to listen to myself and do what I need. If I need to sleep in, that's fine. If I want chocolate, that's also fine.

"It's always amusing to me now when people talk to me about their different diets, whether it be low-carb, Paleo, or something else. I remember when I used to be in that phase. So focused on controlling everything: my meals, my exercise, the right amount of calories. I felt good, until something went wrong in my plan. I may not look exactly as I want to yet, but the majority of the stress of sticking to a certain plan and having to follow something specific is gone. I still continue to lose weight but can do so while also eating what I want.

"People are always talking, trying to figure out the secret to weight loss. But in reality it's not about all of the things you can't have. It's not about figuring out the rules and then just abiding by them to lose weight, because, in reality, every day is different. My schedule, hunger levels, and mood vary daily. Sometimes I want to go out for Italian, but other times I'm tired and just want to heat up a frozen meal. Sometimes I'm stressed and have the energy and desire to attend a spin class, but other days I'm exhausted and all I want is to go to bed. How can I not have flexibility with my food and exercise plan when every day for me isn't the same? So if you're looking for the secret to weight loss, don't ask someone else what you should be doing; ask yourself. The rest will fall in line."

ACKNOWLEDGMENTS

I never quite understood Hillary Rodham Clinton's "It takes a village to raise a child" until writing this book. Well, it takes a village to write a book and raise children simultaneously. My village encompasses four types of people: my editors and contributors, my family, my friends, and my clients.

I would first like to acknowledge and thank Anne Egan, editorial director of Rodale Direct Books, for recommending me for this project. My thanks go out to the Rodale staff members, including Jeff Csatari, Gillian Francella, Nancy Bailey, Hope Clarke, and Chris Krogermeier, who helped me transform science into everyday English so that all women may understand their bodies and change their relationship with food. Deep gratitude to all who shared their wisdom, including but not limited to Dr. Ralph Carson of Fit Rx; Dr. Anita Johnston, author of *Eating in the Light of the Moon;* and my certified eating disorder specialists, the IAEDP NY crew—Susan Schrott, LCSW, CEDS, and Kripalu-certified yoga instructor; Adrienne Glasser, LCSW, RDMT, creator of Active Insight; and Maria Sorbara Mora, MS, CEDRD, PRYT, RYT. Biggest hugs and thanks to Laura Iu, RD, of DoWhatIuLove.com. Your friendship, support since 2012, and now endless help with recipe development and testing for this book are unparalleled.

And, of course, thank you to my village. I could not have written this book without the tireless help of my parents, Joan and Richard; my sister, Janine; my husband, Robert; and my in-laws, Ginny and Bob, who cared for my two boys during the creation of this book. Thank you to the two best people and things in my life, Robert and William. I hope my career will one day inspire your own dreams (and, of course, your respect for women).

Mom, you asked me to write a book. Well, here is my third. Thank you, Mom and Dad, for always believing in me and teaching me the American Dream is possible.

Thank you to my best friends, who motivate, guide, and support my every effort. I would never have pushed so hard and far without you and your professional advice: Liza Boyd Benson, Kelly Arcella, Jaime Hollander, Sara Garlick (and

Lin, too). A special thank-you to my friends and colleagues who shape the way I counsel my clients: Jennifer G of Jen G Yoga; Elyse Falk, RD; Dr. Elissa Zelman, CEDS; Jessica Aronson, LCSW, CEDS; and Dr. Mittsi Crossman, CEDS.

Last but not least my most sincere gratitude goes to my clients. AW, CS, JH, MB, and DS, with whom I've spent much of my time over the past years, you inspire and shape me. Most of all, I am grateful for all the tears and laughs we have shared together. To all my clients who have contributed to this book: Wow, thank you. Thank you for choosing me as your RD and thank you for believing in our work. Your success makes every day of my career more worthy than you can imagine. Thank you for sharing your secrets and successes with the readers of this book. Women's honesty and courage to face their relationships with food-body-mind are nothing less than honorable. I am forever grateful to you. All of you truly affect my every day and every way in which I counsel and treat others.

Thank you to my village. I love, respect, and feel the utmost gratitude toward you. This book would not be possible without all of you. Hugs and smiles.

INDEX